P9-BZE-788

# DISCARD

# Challenging Conceptions

## Pregnancy and Parenting Beyond the Traditional Family

*Lisa Saffron*

CASSELL

Cassell
Villiers House, 41/47 Strand
London WC2N 5JE

387 Park Avenue South
New York, NY 10016–8810

First published 1994

**British Library Cataloguing-in-Publication Data**
A catalogue record for this book is available from the British
Library.

**Library of Congress Cataloging-in-Publication Data**
Available from the Library of Congress.

ISBN  0–304–33078–7 (hardback)
       0–304–33076–0 (paperback)

Typeset by Fakenham Photosetting Ltd, Fakenham, Norfolk
Printed and bound in Great Britain by
Mackays of Chatham PLC

# Contents

# *Preface*

I FIRST considered the idea of becoming a mother shortly after meeting lesbian mothers who had done self-insemination. It has been important to me to know that I am part of a growing community of women consciously choosing to have children without men. In 1986 when my self-inseminated baby was nearly a year old, I wrote *Getting Pregnant Our Own Way*. I wrote *Challenging Conceptions* when my child was seven. I want to encourage those lesbians and single women hovering on the brink of motherhood to know that they are not alone, that their desire to have a child can be realized and that there is a wealth of parenting experience to be shared. By writing this book, I aim to make our experience of self-insemination more visible, and in the process to validate, for ourselves and others, the rights of lesbians to be mothers.

I am especially grateful to all the women, men and children I interviewed for the book. They willingly and honestly shared their experiences so that other women can benefit.

Many women made valuable contributions to this book by reading and criticizing the drafts. I would particularly like to thank the following for their help: Marge Berer, Charmaine Brouard, Gill Butler, Da Choong of the Terrence Higgins Trust, Sally Collings, Barbara James, Maria Kennedy, Sheila Mcdonald, Sheila McWattie, Cheri Pies, Jill Radford of Rights of Women, Dena Saffron, members of a lesbian self-insemination group, Joan Walsh, Ruth Wallsgrove, Patricia Wejr, and Women's Health in London.

# Introduction

● *Judy (1986)*

*I'd always wanted a child. I've been a lesbian for six or seven years. In my opinion there were no alternatives. I couldn't adopt. I didn't want to have sex with a man. I wanted to share getting pregnant with my lover Kath. Self-insemination was my only choice. I'm glad I didn't go to a clinic for AID because self-insemination was in our control. The donor was more likely to be someone I'd want as a donor (a politically sussed Jewish gay man rather than a white gentile medical student). The experience was good, the procedure straightforward and not medicalized. We did it, not medical staff. I feel it was the only and right thing for me to do.*

Self-insemination (SI) is a way for fertile women to get pregnant without sexual contact with a man and without medical intervention. It is technically very simple, needing no training and no medical equipment. The procedure is so simple that it can be explained in one page, but the social and political consequences of self-insemination are what fill this book.

Most of the women who consider and practise self-insemination are lesbians, but there are also a smaller number of single heterosexual women. This book is written for all these women, with an emphasis on the experience of lesbians. It gives a mixture of practical advice and personal experiences to explore the many issues raised by choosing self-insemination. It is intended not only as a guide to help women with the mechanics of getting pregnant but as a way of sharing experiences of the consequences of self-insemination – parenting and co-parenting, single parenting, splitting up and staying together, relationships (or none) with donors, communicating with the children, not getting pregnant, telling others, the risk of infection and disease, and the legal position of all the people involved.

# What this book covers

The book starts with a chapter on donors. In the section 'Anonymous or known?', women share their experiences of deciding on the type of contact they wanted with a donor and how they found the right man. I interviewed four men who have been donors, whose accounts appear throughout the book, with the section here focusing specifically on their reasons for and their experiences of being donors ('Being a donor'). An appendix explains what self-insemination is all about and what is required of men should they agree to be donors (Appendix B, 'Advice for Donors about Self-insemination'). This can be photocopied and given to men who are asked to be a donor.

Chapter 2, 'Screening', includes up-to-date information on the risks of HIV and other sexually transmitted diseases, as well as guidelines for checking your own state of health. There is a sample questionnaire for donors in Appendix C.

In Chapter 3, 'Getting Pregnant', you are guided through the four steps to getting pregnant. Step 1 is about how to identify when you are fertile. Step 2 is getting the donor to ejaculate and then taking simple measures to keep the sperm alive for up to eight hours until you can do Step 3 – inseminating during your fertile days and at least twice in a cycle. Finally, Step 4 is the two-week wait.

Many women doing self-insemination start off or end up doing it on their own, and their experiences are covered in 'Doing it on your own' in Chapter 4. In 'Doing it together', the experiences of co-parents or non-biological mothers are made visible. The perspectives of co-parents appear alongside those of biological mothers in many sections throughout the book, but this one focuses on the issues for women in couples.

As a result of years of lesbian parenting, I have been able to bring in the children's experiences in Chapter 5. 'Communicating with children' is a section with full accounts of children's reactions and mothers' experiences of explaining to their children about self-insemination, about being lesbian, about donors and about different kinds of family. In the section 'A few words from the children', a 12-year-old boy and girl tell what it has been like for them.

Three significant new laws have been passed in the last few years. In Chapter 6, 'The Law', I explain what we need to know about the Children Act 1989 and the Child Support Act 1992. The Children Act has made major changes to the rights of the donor, and potentially to those of the co-parent, while the Child Support Act affects those women claiming benefits. The Human Fertilization and Embryology Act 1990 is explained in Chapter 9, 'Donor Insemination through Clinics' (see below). It has not affected the legal position of self-insemination but is important in its influence on clinics offering donor insemination. It is still too early for there to be any test cases, which would give us an idea of how these laws will be interpreted.

Sadly, self-insemination does not always lead to a baby, or it may take many months or years of trying before success. The experiences of those women who have done self-insemination but did not get pregnant or who are still trying are as much a part of the process as the experiences of those who now have children. Their voices are heard in Chapter 7, 'When SI Isn't Working'.

Having a child is such a public matter that telling others can't be avoided. The strategies and experiences of women telling their family, friends and doctors are covered in Chapter 8, 'Telling Others'.

Although this book is primarily about self-insemination, I have put in a chapter on 'Donor Insemination through Clinics' (Chapter 9) as this is still a valid option for lesbians and single women. The British Pregnancy Advisory Service used to offer donor insemination to lesbians and single women at a number of its clinics throughout England, but closed its service in July 1991, significantly restricting women's options throughout Britain. However, there are other clinics which do not discriminate against lesbians and single women.

Resources and further reading are listed in Appendix A.

This book is about getting pregnant but it's not a pregnancy book. It doesn't attempt to cover the experience of pregnancy or your childbirth options, or to prepare you for possible tragedies such as stillbirths and cot deaths. There are many other books available on these subjects which are relevant to any woman getting pregnant. This book focuses on what is specific to lesbians and single women having children by donor insemination.

For this book, thirty-three people contributed their personal experiences. Eighteen of them appeared in *Getting Pregnant Our Own Way*, the first version of this book, which was published in

1986. Seven of these women were re-interviewed to give their perspectives six years on. Except for the children's stories, each person's account is divided up, with sections in different chapters. If you want to follow one person's story, you can trace it through the index. The date at the beginning of each account is the time when the person was interviewed or wrote the piece. All the names are pseudonyms.

These accounts are snapshots of a moment in time. They are not stories with a beginning, middle and end or even a clear plot. Each story is simply the way that woman perceived events or how she wanted to present herself at the time I interviewed her.

# Creating our own families

Lesbians and single women are under attack for our choice to have children. It is not surprising that women often feel defensive, or under pressure to be 'good mothers' or to present themselves as having the 'perfect family'. Women spoke about their anxiety that they were not living up to some undisclosed expectation. Some apologized for doing it differently from their idea of the lesbian 'norm'. There was worry that the painful times meant they were doing something wrong. Women were aware of the consequences of choosing to go against the grain – that we are unlikely to get any sympathy if we run into difficulties later. Some women were concerned about the impact of exposing our lives publicly to those outside the lesbian community, fearing that honesty about painful experiences would show lesbians in a poor light. Many of the women I interviewed struggled with these pressures.

Sharing our personal experiences is one way of making our lives as lesbian mothers visible, of validating our choices and of learning from each other. It is important for all of us to know that there are other women doing self-insemination. The women interviewed for this book, as well as the children and the men, are not necessarily typical of all people doing self-insemination, yet they represent a wide range of experiences. I want to convey that there are as many ways to go about this as there are individuals doing it and that each of us is creating our own future.

There is no formula for successful family making and very few role models of lesbian parents or of single mothers by choice. There is no right way to do it. It is not more right-on to have an anonymous donor than a known donor or two lesbian mothers rather than one, or vice versa. We are part of a lesbian community which is very diverse, with women making widely differing choices about the kind of family they create. This diversity is something to celebrate and honour. We live in a society that passively denies or actively attacks the rights of lesbian-led families to exist. The courage and strength we have to live our lives as we choose comes from each other – from knowing there are other lesbians having children and from acceptance of each other's struggles.

The existence of lesbian and single mothers is a threat to traditional family values. Consciously or not, we are challenging the need for fathers, the institution of marriage and the male–female couple as the model of the ideal parents. We are saying that families can be made up of different people with a variety of relationships to each other and still be healthy places in which children can grow up and in which women can be mothers. We are changing the basic definition of a family. No longer is it limited to a group of people related by blood, marriage or divorce. We are expanding it to include a group of people who love and care for each other. It doesn't even have to include children. Our families are not lacking in anything. There is no need to compensate for the absence of a father or to apologize for not conforming to the expected family norm.

This book presents no justification of lesbian and single motherhood, since none is necessary. It starts with the assumption that women are going ahead, despite society's prejudices towards our methods of conception, the families we create, our lesbianism or our ability to be good mothers. As more babies are being born and our children grow up, we too are growing up into greater acceptance of ourselves as lesbian and single mothers.

## ● *Laura (1992)*

*I think of her conception as a private event, a secret, a miracle ... and I don't want to talk about it. It was magic. Such strong magic that we, as women, can take this simple, strong stuff called semen, take it literally in our hands, deliver it to our bodies, and by this act conceive children. So, I don't want to get into talk that equates this extraordinary but simple, powerful but simple, miraculous act (in the sense that the creation of life is a miracle) with mere mechanics, as if donors were a kind of medical achieve-*

*ment, as if transferring sperm from one place to another were something new, highly technical, scientific and difficult, which for the most part, it isn't. It could quite easily have been done throughout the ages once people knew that sperm and women's bodies produced children (sometimes)!*

# Chapter one

# Donors

## Anonymous or known?

UNLIKE donor insemination through a clinic, self-insemination potentially allows a woman to choose the type of contact she wants with a donor. I have categorized these into four main types:

1. anonymous donor;
2. known identity but no contact;
3. known identity with contact;
4. co-parenting donor.

To make the decision, a woman has to take into account the feelings of several people – herself as the biological mother, her partner if she has one, the child and the donor. Once a woman has agreed with her partner or by herself how she feels about contact or not with a donor and has thought what is best for the child, she can then set about finding a man who will fit in. In theory, the decision about what kind of contact you want influences how you go about finding a donor. In practice, the process of finding a donor sometimes determines what kind of donor you end up with. That is why it is so important to decide first what you want and then compromise if you have to.

### Finding a donor

Once a woman has decided whether she wants a known or an anonymous donor, she then has to find a man who will cooperate. This is rarely an easy matter and many women pursue a number of possibilities before they find one that works. They ask male friends, friends of friends, brothers of lovers, former lovers and men in men's groups. They advertise in magazines such as *Time Out* in London or the *Pink Paper* nationally. They ask women who have done self-insemination if they can use their donors. They may form groups for mutual support, helping each other find donors and providing much-needed encouragement and support. Some groups compile a register of donors, interviewing them and screening them for the group as a whole and then offering individual members of the group the chance to choose the donor who meets their requirements. It is not necessarily easier for a group to find donors than for an individual woman. It may even be harder, as some men may feel more comfortable responding to an ad if they think that means they will know the woman they will be doing a favour for.

Men willing to be donors are more often found in social circles where it is acceptable for lesbians and single women to have children. In communities where this is not a common practice, women may have a harder task. There are no absolute guidelines on how to find a donor. It is really a matter of pursuing any contacts available to you as well as getting people to ask on your behalf.

## Anonymous donors

Women who want the donor to be anonymous are making this decision because they feel that the biological father's presence is irrelevant to the family they are creating. This is the same point of view taken by male–female couples who get help from a clinic when the male partner is infertile. In these couples, it is the male partner who will be the father regardless of his biological ties to the child. In the families created by lesbian couples and single women, the anonymous donor has no further role once he has made pregnancy possible.

Women without male partners often choose anonymous donors because of fear that a donor may change his mind at some time in the future about his parenting role. (See Chapter 6, 'The Law'.) Lesbian mothers are vulnerable to losing their children in custody cases. Too close an involvement with their child's biological father could make them feel at risk.

For a donor to be anonymous, women usually use intermediaries who know how to contact the donor and who make all the arrangements. This tends to involve frequent negotiations, and arrangements can be complicated and sometimes frustrating. The intermediary has to be trusted not to reveal the identities to anyone at the time of the inseminations as well as in the future. This puts her in a difficult position of power.

A woman may preserve the donor's anonymity yet still make it possible for the child to trace him by making a special agreement with the donor. A reliable person such as a solicitor can hold information about the donor's identity and current address, and agree to release it only to the child.

## Known donors

My impression is that there is a trend towards more women choosing to know the donor's identity rather than having anonymous donors. Many women do not want the donor to be in the role of a social father yet want to know his identity and sometimes to meet him, usually for the sake of the child. Some women take this position because they do not feel strongly enough to make the effort to ensure anonymity or are not convinced that the donor poses a legal threat. They may be put off by the complicated arrangements needed for the donor to remain anonymous. The desire to know what the donor looks like is quite common. Women may want to know the donor so as to have an image of him as a real person, rather than being totally unknown.

The type of contact may be negotiated early on, or may develop naturally as the woman and man get to know each other, or may be initiated by the child. Encouraging contact carries certain risks as well as satisfying the children's interest in their biological father. Although the donor does not automatically have parental responsibility, he can apply to court to acquire it under the Children Act. Any contact that he has had with the child will strengthen his case and it will appear in the eyes of the court that it was your intention for him to be the child's father. See Chapter 6, 'The Law', for a fuller discussion of the legal position of the donor.

Co-parenting with a man is one reason women give for choosing a known donor. Women who want to co-parent with the donor usually make arrangements with a close male friend, but some advertise for men willing to co-parent with them. They negotiate the level of involvement and decide together whether the donor will play a father role or will be more of an 'uncle' figure. With strangers, there is always the possibility that the relationships will change as the donor ceases to be a stranger and as parenting creates new challenges. Even friendships of long standing will be changed by the demands of co-parenting a growing child. The friendship may be strengthened by the experience, or challenged.

## The issues for the child

Do the children conceived by self-insemination have a right to know their biological origins? Should women make sure they know the identity of the donor for the child's sake even if they want no contact with him? The issues for the child are inevitably different from those for the mother, but it is not always possible to predict how a child will feel. Many children do want to know who their father is, but not all. Some show no curiosity or are only mildly interested. Some ask and are satisfied with the answer. Yet it is probably too soon to generalize about what the children want, as the oldest children conceived by self-insemination are still in their early teens. We don't know how they will feel when they reach adulthood and start having children of their own.

On one level, it does seem strange for children to attach value to a relationship with a person they have never met and who plays no significant role in their everyday life. Perhaps one day society's attitudes on the importance of the blood relationship will change. But whether the desire to know one's genetic roots is socially induced or not, it is true that the desire is there in many children who have been conceived by donor insemination, in the same way it is in children who have been adopted. It may conflict with what the mother wants but for many, if not most, children, there is a desire to know who their biological father is.

By choosing an anonymous donor, the mother is making a decision for her child that cannot necessarily be reversed. It may be difficult to trace the man if the child wants to meet him, though it is unlikely to be impossible. It is usually too complicated to arrange true anonymity and there is inevitably someone who has a lead. There can never be the guarantee of total anonymity with self-insemination that there is by having donor insemination at a clinic, though it is probably adequate for what women want. Some women feel that not knowing the donor's identity makes it easier for the mother to tell her children that she doesn't know who he is, thus indicating very clearly that he has no role in the family.

Depending on the child, this may or may not turn out to be an easy decision to live with.

Some women meet the donor and keep in contact so that they can tell the child who he is and something about him, if or when the child should ask. Children can then make their own decision to get to know him, if they want to. Knowing the donor's identity means there is always the possibility of making contact. It need never be acted upon, but the option is there. If children do ask to meet the donors, the mothers have a choice of how to respond.

## The issues for donors

Women who want anonymous donors are looking for men who are prepared to give up any interest they might have had in their offspring. The men are asked to have the same feelings about donating sperm as they would about giving blood. They are doing a favour to women they do not know, but the men themselves can expect no emotional or practical involvement in the outcome. There are men willing to be donors on these terms.

Women who want the donors to have contact are entering unfamiliar territory, requiring soul-searching and clear communication on everyone's part. The men must ask themselves how they will feel about being contacted at some time in the future. This is understandably difficult to answer, because they are unlikely to have been in this circumstance before and cannot easily predict how they will feel in a situation which is hypothetical and unusual. They need to satisfy themselves that they will not be asked to take on parental responsibility. Many men are willing to be contacted by the child and are open to whatever develops.

## Developing contact between donor and child

Children have asked to meet donors and there have been examples where this has been arranged. In this situation, they are embarking on a new set of relationships with few role models of how to proceed. It may be initiated by the child, but the mother and the donor are participants with their own desires and feelings. While being open to what may develop, the adults must clarify to each other what they want to happen. They may be looking to set up a one-off meeting or they may want ongoing contact. There are issues to consider about how far to let the relationship develop and what names to use to describe those relationships.

### ● *Mary (1986)*

*In 1979 I was a member of a lesbian self-insemination group. We tried to get donors by asking heterosexual feminists. Most heterosexual women were appalled by the idea. There were at least a couple of occasions on which the men, for whatever reasons, would have been quite happy to give sperm, but their girlfriends just couldn't bear the thought of their man's sperm being used to bring about a child. That certainly made me feel very bitter about the support we could expect from heterosexual women. It was a lesbian who helped us find our donors, and the donors that we did find were gay men.*

### ● *Sheila (1992)*

*As soon as I learned that it was a possibility, I decided I wanted to have an anonymous donor rather than pick up a strange man and sleep with him. There were a number of reasons for choosing an anonymous donor. I knew that sleeping with a man could never be a neutral experience for me. If I did get a baby out of it, then I might have ended up with lovely feelings about the man or I might have wanted to have more contact with him. If it turned out to be a horrible experience, I wouldn't want that to be the start of my child. I always felt that I didn't want to make a long-term commitment to someone for all those years, whether to a man or to a woman. It seemed to me that that's what I would be doing if I knew the man. Tying us to someone else was just not what I had in mind for me and my child. I felt that it was better not to have a father than to have a vague, shadowy figure, some hazy memory. Doing it by an anonymous donor was more neutral.*

*In 1978, there was a big shock-horror scandal in the papers because the* Evening News *had exposed the fact that lesbians were going to a doctor in Harley Street and getting donors from him. At that point I was definitely thinking about having a baby, but I only knew how to get pregnant by the traditional method. So the* Evening News *opened up another possibility. I actually went to that doctor once and did it. I got his name from Sappho [a lesbian organization]. He gave me a five-minute interview during which he* told me to work out for myself when I ovulate and come along when I was ready. When I did go along, I was given the sperm in a little plastic vial inside a brown envelope. I don't even remember being given any advice about keeping it warm or having to hurry home. We went in a pub and I put it down my bra to keep it warm and then went home and did the insemination.

Having done that once, I realized that it was crazy going to a doctor. All I needed was to find a man and do it myself. Just when I was thinking that, I saw an ad in the London Women's Liberation Newsletter *advertising a group for lesbians who were thinking about getting pregnant [the same group Mary was in]. I answered the ad and six of us started meeting and talking about it. Most of us had already tried some way or other. Very soon after we started meeting, we began thinking about ways of finding men. The obvious way at the time was to think about gay men. Through a friend of a friend, we heard of a gay men's consciousness-raising group. We asked them to talk in their group about being donors for us. The answer came back that they would do it. We set up a dinner for some of the women and some of the men to talk about the practicalities and what we wanted from the arrangement – to make sure there were no misunderstandings.

We set it up so that whenever we needed the sperm, we rang up a man who took responsibility for that task for a couple of months, until someone else took over. That man would phone round all the blokes, sort out who would do it for us, then ring us back to tell us where to go and when to pick it up. The first few times I did it, I arranged for somebody to go and pick it up for me. We were really careful about keeping it all anonymous. By about the third month, it didn't seem important any more not to know where the donor's house was. We started to go to their houses and do the inseminations there. That was much nicer than having to drag all the way back again, especially as I couldn't always find someone to go and get it for me. It seemed easier to just go there, do it in the room, lie down for a few minutes, and then go away. I did get a glimpse of the men, but it was a different man on each occasion, so I only have vague memories of what they looked like. I couldn't distinguish which one it was that gave me the sperm to get pregnant.

Fourteen years later and with a 12-year-old son, I feel confirmed that the decision to use an anonymous donor was right for me and Tim. The way Tim and I always talk about it is that he *doesn't have a father. We talk about the story quite often. He knows the exact details. I don't want to say that I haven't questioned it but I don't think anything has ever led me to feel that I wish I had done it differently.*

### ● *Judy (1986)*

The self-insemination group that I was a member of was formed after ads in the London Women's Liberation Newsletter [not the same group as Mary and Sheila's]. There were about four or five of us meeting regularly over a year or more. The donors were found through other women who wanted to do SI or through friends. I asked a couple of men I knew. One was excluded because he'd had hepatitis; another was reluctant because he'd not sorted out how he felt; another was interested and had been screened before [had a sperm count] and was used by other women who I don't know directly. They were all men I liked and trusted and I would have been happy to have as donors, except that I knew them and didn't want their involvement with the baby to be connected with 'biological fathering'. I think it should be emphasized that men are reluctant to be donors and the majority of those that do, do it because of political reasons – i.e. to support lesbians. Most of them are gay, as was the one of my friends who agreed.

We began setting up a donor network before the AIDS problem exploded so this didn't enter into our discussions. A gay bloke I asked to be a donor later for someone else, when I was already pregnant, declined partly on the grounds of AIDS. He didn't know if he was HIV-positive or not. We talked in the group not so much about the sexuality of donors as the number of partners and degree of sexual activity. Either gay or straight men who were very sexually active would be more likely to have had a sexually transmitted disease.

My lover, Kath, and I found my donor through women friends. I wanted him to be totally anonymous because I didn't want any comeback at a later date in terms of the donor wanting access [to the child]. I wanted to be in control of the situation. I went through a lot of heart-searching about this and talked to other women. Two women friends who are heterosexual single mothers were really supportive and encouraging (more so than some lesbian friends). At one point I thought it would be better if I knew the donor but he didn't know me. Then I decided I didn't want to live *with the information. I can always in truth say, 'I don't know who the father is.' I think it's a hard decision to make and I worry whether my child will understand why I made it.*

### ● Kath (1986)

*It was very important to me that Judy's donor was anonymous because I didn't want to have to confront at any point some kind of threat or challenge from a person who had no other connection with us apart from being the donor.*

*We spent two years in the self-insemination group. That was great – having the opportunity to talk. It gave us the feeling that we weren't all by ourselves. I feel that it's a really good idea to set up groups for support. We talked about everything – why children, when, in what kind of situations, all the issues around donors, all that. It helped me a lot.*

### ● Cathy (1986)

*At first I had something against doing self-insemination. I was worried that something in the process could damage the sperm. I preferred the 'natural' method – knowing face to face who the father was. The easiest, most obvious thing was to use a man who I was friends with. I didn't actually know any other men. I did ask him but he didn't want to be a father. I didn't want to go out in the street and grab a man. I finally came to the conclusion that self-insemination was the only way I was going to get pregnant. So I started asking around for donors. It took quite a few months and I was getting more desperate as time went on. Once you decide you want to be pregnant, then you want to be pregnant that second. I didn't really talk to my lover, Jean, about it or involve her in finding donors. It was my private search. I talked to women at work who were pregnant and in unconventional relationships. I was given Diane's phone number by two different people. Eventually I went to see her and she said she'd help me use some gay men she knew. So I set up times to go and inseminate.*

*I used two men which could have meant that I wouldn't know who the father was. That worried me a little bit but didn't stop me. I was just desperate to have a child. Since then, I've come to think it's important to know who the father is. My daughter looks like one of the men, who has very distinctive features. I knew him because he lived in the same house as Diane. I couldn't have used an anonymous donor.*

### ● Jean (1986)

*When I decided I wanted to get pregnant, I wanted to do it that very month. I had organized an insemination with a donor and had been quite careful about it. But I didn't inseminate because the donor said his ex-lover was HIV-positive and was very sick. I then decided to ask the only other man that I was close to and knew quite well – my lover Cathy's cousin. But that was a no-go area because it would have caused too many ripples in a network of friendships, so I had to start the search for a donor.*

*I finally found my 'perfect' donor after advertising in the small ads of City Limits. I got seven replies. All, except one, were genuine and generous offers to help that really surprised me as, up until then, I'd always associated small ads and lonely hearts with loonies, and it was only because all other sources of donors had dried up that I was driven to advertise. Cathy wrote a long letter to the man we chose, explaining who we were and what we wanted, and put our phone number only as a contact. He phoned us and agreed to help. The first time he donated sperm, we arranged to do it at a friend's house. Cathy chatted to him, briefly reiterating that I did want him to be known to the child. I felt very strongly that I wanted my child to be able to know who their father was if he or she wanted to. I don't feel that I could deliberately deprive them of that knowledge. After that first meeting, Cathy said that he appeared to be a perfectly ordinary nice young man, so we arranged for him to visit our house. I was very curious to meet him and luckily it was easy and relaxed. It's very important to me to know as much as I can about the donor – his health, family background, ideas and politics, and for him to see me and Cathy in a long-term, steady relationship, already with one child. However, he completely freaked out about what he'd done after Elaine was born and changed his mind about having any contact with us. [See Jean's piece in 'Communicating with children', Chapter 5.]*

### ● Eunice (1992)

*The first donor Stella and I found was a work colleague of a friend, and although he never met Stella, I interviewed him with one of the other women from the SI group. He was quite young with a good head of hair, an important criterion when selecting a donor, and was initially very cooperative. He agreed to all the health checks that we asked for, so there was only the delay of waiting for the test results. This was really nerve-wracking, as we kept thinking that, having more time to think about it, he'd change his mind, or that there would be a problem with the test results – in fact we pretty much covered everything that could go wrong. Nothing did go wrong, and this donor remained with us for six months.*

*We had joined a lesbian SI group and were working on getting a 'back-up' donor in case the present one dropped out. We'd had an idea that this might happen when, despite all the information we'd given him, he expressed surprise that Stella hadn't got pregnant on the first attempt. We eventually advertised and met with some of the potential donors but this didn't really work out, until another group member put us in touch with someone who had replied to their advert and whom they had interviewed. This time Stella met him by herself, as I'd managed to convince myself, after several unsuccessful meetings with potential donors, that together we were probably rather overwhelming. This time we were lucky and the donor turned out to be the sort of person we were looking for. He was prepared to donate without wanting anything further in terms of contact with a child, and his requests were reasonable. After successful medical checks we started inseminating and Stella fell pregnant on the seventh attempt.*

*It took two donors and eighteen months before Stella got pregnant. During this time our views on contact with donors changed slightly. Initially the idea was for total anonymity, with 'runners' meeting the donor and doing the collections. The first donor knew very little about us, and claimed that he wasn't particularly bothered as long as he was told when/if Stella got pregnant. I was probably happier with this than Stella was, because as time went on Stella started to feel more and more that we ought to be able to allow a child some element of choice in finding out about the donor when they were older. This was obviously something that the donor would have to agree to, and I felt reluctant to let some other person have this as yet undefined possible future relationship with our child. For some time I was positively indignant, but was eventually convinced, once I stopped thinking about my own position and imagined it from the child's point of view (this actually took longer than one might imagine).*

*The main thing is that if I'd had my way, there would be no going back and our child would have been stuck with that decision. We now have a son named Robert and although we've met the donor and know quite a bit about him, he doesn't have detailed information about us. We've agreed that although there is to be no planned contact, he will notify us of his whereabouts over the years via a solicitor in case Robert feels that he wants to contact him in the future. The donor feels that he will not have children of his own, and says he would be happy with this arrangement even if he did. His main request from us was that we let him have a photograph of Robert when he was born, but now that this has happened, he has gone to great lengths to provide us with information and photos of his own family. We were for a time very worried that despite having been clear with him, he may decide that he wants more contact. As lesbians, we are very aware of our weak position in law. However, we have since been reassured about his motives and he is now actively seeking other women to act as donor.*

● Paula (1991)

*I knew that I didn't want a donor to be involved with my child and I think my girlfriend Nicole was quite happy about that. At one point I thought I would have been happy to have some involvement if I had known any men, but she was always much more keen on non-involvement. As it happened the man didn't want to be involved. So it was never an issue. There has been indirect contact through our go-between. If Tara wants to know who he is, he's quite happy to have some sort of contact. I feel quite happy about that. He won't be considered to be a parent. She has said daddy a few times and I've just said, 'You haven't got one'. I haven't thought about it very much.*

● Shaheen (1992)

*I wanted an anonymous donor. If I had had a male friend that I had known for years and who I got on with OK and could trust, then maybe I would have asked him. Because I didn't know any men like that, I wanted the donor to be anonymous. I couldn't live with the worry hanging over me that the man could appear at any stage and claim his child. Every knock at the door would make me tense.*

I did self-insemination. I had heard of women going through clinics and trying for a very long time, spending large sums of money and not getting anywhere. It seemed that fresh sperm worked a lot quicker than frozen sperm, so I decided to pursue my own donor.

First of all, I asked around friends of mine if they knew of any men who would be willing. No one came up with anything. We decided that I'd give my partner Jackie's donor a go. She had got the name of a man who lived not far away from us from a self-insemination group. She tried SI with him and she also went to a clinic because her cycle was completely bizarre. She couldn't work out any regularity to it. It took her a while to get pregnant and then she miscarried very early on and decided not to try any more. I tried with him for five months. He was very good but I didn't conceive. I knew when I ovulated because I had done my charts for six months beforehand. I was getting panicky by this time.

Someone suggested I try another donor. That's when I put an ad in City Limits. I did get quite a few responses but they weren't any good. They were either men whose sperm was too sacred to put in a jam jar and just didn't want anything to do with SI or men who really didn't know what they were letting themselves in for. I didn't want to see any of them. I wanted it to be anonymous. Jackie wanted to meet them to see if they were OK health-wise and to check out their motives. She met one man. He seemed OK but he let me down at the last minute, so we had to give that one a miss.

Then we decided to ask around our friends again. A friend of Jackie's who is a social worker put it around her colleagues at her area office. She came up with someone she worked with and who is a close friend of hers. He had a partner who he'd been with for about ten years and who was willing for him to be a donor. I conceived the first time I inseminated with him.

I know the donor's name and where he lives. I have photographs of him. But he doesn't know who I am. He only knows that I conceived.

● Hazel (1991)

The donor is a friend of a friend. He actually approached my friend, saying in conversation that he wouldn't mind leaving a bit of himself behind. She said, 'Have I got a woman for you!' She phoned us up and told us that she thought this guy might be interested in *being a donor. We met him at her house. Everything was done at her house. We don't know where he lives. We met him, had dinner together, chatted about what we wanted out of this deal. His lover (a man) doesn't know anything about it so he didn't want any involvement and we didn't want him involved at all. He had been tested [for HIV] and he was clear. He tested again for us before we got together again.*

*We saw him at my friend's flat twice for the inseminations. He made the donation and went off to his aerobics class. Donna and I stayed around and I inseminated. We arranged to meet again the next month, but because it worked the first time, I never saw him again. He heard through my friend that it had worked and that we didn't need him any more. When Jordan was born, Donna phoned him and left him a message at work saying that Jordan had been born and that he was healthy. He phoned back and said that that's great and that he wouldn't mind a photograph every now and again. He also said he wouldn't mind if Jordan looked him up when Jordan was older. But he didn't want to play a father role. Because he's keeping it a secret, I can't imagine that he would cause any trouble so I'm not frightened about it at all. I wouldn't know him on the street. We'll never bump into him. I'm not concerned about him wanting to get more involved later on.*

● *Jill (1992)*

*The whole issue about the anonymity of the donor has come up for me in a big way recently, because I'm planning to have my second child and I've given a lot of thought to the matter of the donor. I discussed it early on with my son, Tom, who is nearly 7. He was conceived by self-insemination by an anonymous donor. Tom was absolutely clear about what he wanted. If the baby was going to have a dad around, then he wanted that man to be his dad too. Otherwise he wanted the baby's donor to be anonymous. I started off thinking that I would try and find someone who would have some involvement but, the more I thought about it, the clearer it seemed that anonymity was preferable. Although it has certain problems, it is at least simple and straightforward with no future possibility of any traumas. My great fear of having a donor involved is that I might lose control of the situation. What if he wants to see the child more than I want him to? What if he and I* don't get on and just having him around in our lives at all is a hassle?

But donors are hard to find and I feel I can't be too choosy. I have now found someone who is willing to be a non-anonymous donor. I've explained my situation and he knows that any relationship with the baby involves some relationship with Tom too. At this stage I'm not anticipating that he'll be around very much. I feel safer about this guy because he's the brother of a friend who thinks very highly of him, and also because he is in a long-term relationship with a woman and so the child will presumably not be the major focus of his attention. I still feel a bit scared about what I'm letting myself in for, though.

The arrangement we've made regarding future contact between him and the child is for them to meet when s/he starts asking about him and then we'll just take it from there. I feel fine about that and am much less concerned about what might happen in the future than I was. I thought Tom might be disappointed that he wasn't going to see this man regularly, but in fact, his major concern was that he shouldn't be left out of any contact that does happen. Only time will tell, of course, whether my struggles have produced a workable solution or not. At this point, I feel reasonably optimistic that it will all turn out well.

### ● Toni (1992)

I started off trying to get pregnant by anonymous donors but eventually got pregnant by self-insemination with a man I met through my girlfriend at the time. The original agreement we made was that he would only be a donor and would have no contact with the child. Now, eight years later, he has become a close friend of mine and a daddy to our daughter, though one without any parental responsibility. Parenting is my activity with the help of Claire's other two mothers. Our relationship with this donor/daddy/friend has developed quite naturally. Looking back, I find it amazing that it has worked out so well when I was so unclear about what I wanted in the beginning.

I was first introduced to self-insemination in 1981, when every lesbian I knew with children had used anonymous donors. A couple of years later, I decided to get pregnant myself. I wasn't interested in finding a man to be a co-parent but I felt the measures they had gone to to assure anonymity were unnecessary and based on more mistrust of men than I felt was warranted. Still, anonymous donors seemed to be the way you did self-insemination at that time and I didn't have strong enough feelings about it to find another way. I soon found myself involved in the most complicated and messy arrangements to get the sperm without meeting the donors. After a few months of this charade, I realized that I felt uncomfortable with the arrangement and that it was unlikely to succeed.

My lover asked a gay couple she knew if they would be willing to be donors for me. They both agreed and we went to their house to talk it over. I don't remember having a very deep discussion about what was involved. They were happy to donate sperm for me and didn't seem to want any contact with the child or any kind of relationship with me. I really appreciate how flexible, accommodating and pleasant they both were. They made themselves totally available, even cancelling other arrangements when I needed them. I was pleased to have found a stress-free and enjoyable way to do the inseminations, and pleased to know who the donors were.

In the month that I conceived, Pierre alone donated sperm, so I had no doubt which was the donor. After Claire was born, I sent Pierre a photo of her and was very disappointed not to hear from him. I assumed that it was of no interest to him and let it drop.

Four years later, in a conversation with a friend of mine, he commented that he knew that he had a daughter and that he would like to see her. This friend was aware of my feelings on the matter and that very night phoned me to relay the information that Pierre was interested in seeing Claire. I wrote to him suggesting that we meet without Claire to discuss what kind of relationship we were embarking on. Knowing that Claire had strong feelings about the concept of 'daddy', I didn't think that a one-off meeting would be enough for her, nor did it feel very satisfying to me. We agreed on regular contact but that he wouldn't take on any parental responsibility.

At this meeting, Pierre told me that he had received the photo I had sent after Claire was born, but had not dared to respond because he felt worried that he would want more contact than had been originally agreed. He also told me that he had recently become infected with the HIV virus. It had occurred long after he had been a donor to me, so neither Claire nor I had been at risk. This diagnosis had influenced Pierre's feelings about seeing

*Claire. He told me that he had always had a fantasy that Claire might contact him when she was 16 or so and wanted to meet her daddy. Since becoming HIV-positive, he was aware that he might not be alive when she becomes old enough to look for him.*

*I felt that we were setting out into uncharted territory. I knew no other lesbians who were introducing the donor to their children. I was aware of hostility from other lesbians who disapproved, or perhaps felt threatened by my choice to let Claire know Pierre as her daddy.*

*At first, it was clear that I was responding to a strong desire on Claire's part to meet her daddy. After several years of asking to see him, she was intensely interested in him when they did meet. But within a few months, the novelty wore off or she was satisfied with what she knew of him. She stopped asking to visit him and didn't seem bothered when I suggested it. Then I became aware that I was organizing visits with Pierre because I wanted to make Pierre happy. It was obvious that he was thrilled to meet his daughter and I wanted him to have a good time with her. She didn't always cooperate and would sometimes ignore him when he came around. I became anxious for his sake that he was pushing her to like him. Every time he came, he brought her presents. I could see that it would backfire and was worried that she would reject him because he was so obviously trying to buy her love. I finally told him not to give her so many presents. I was doing this to protect him, but I did wonder how much I should interfere in their relationship. I became aware of my own needs in this complicated set of interrelationships. Was I trying to make him the kind of father I never had? I found myself caught up in my own unmet childhood needs, projecting them on to Pierre and Claire.*

*In December, Pierre became seriously ill with lymphoma, cancer of the lymph system. This was his first AIDS-related illness, only three years after becoming HIV-positive. He has been given a 50 per cent chance of recovering from the lymphoma. I felt shocked. I had not expected it so soon. More than that, I realized that my grief was not just because Claire might lose a daddy but because I might lose a very good friend. Somehow, without my knowing it, I had become very fond of Pierre. Over the last few months of hospital visits and chemotherapy sessions and concern over what kind of support everyone needs, I have felt very close to Pierre. I stopped focusing on his relationship to Claire. Maybe he did too. Perhaps as a consequence, Claire's basically loving nature was given space to surface. Since his diagnosis with lymphoma, Claire has been natural and relaxed with Pierre, as well as caring and protective of him. She enjoys going to visit him. The awareness of death brings into sharper focus what is really important in life — loving relationships and clear and honest communication. The future of our relationship is still unknown but I am very happy that we took the risk.*

● *Bronwen (1991)*

*The donor I used was the only one available. His partner had suggested it. It was there on offer and since I felt that it was very urgent to get pregnant, I saw it as the only option. At that point, I had just failed to get pregnant by heterosex. The previous year my best friend agreed to do it and then had changed his mind. I had been trying to get hold of donors. There were one or two others, who seemed dodgy.*

*It's not like me not to have everything all worked out, but it is most organic how my son Rhys's and my relationship with the donor and his family has developed. Because I trust the donor and his partner and we share a lot in common, I feel we can handle just about everything. I'm very, very fond of his partner, and trust their values, and love their parenting, and would even consider asking them to have Rhys if anything happened to me and my friend David couldn't have him. This is not because he's the donor but because they are the family whose parenting is closest to mine. At one point a long time ago before I had Rhys, they talked about me having their son if anything happened to them.*

*I'm lucky in retrospect that they are such a great couple and great parents, though I do worry occasionally. He could always go odd, go haywire. If his partner left him and took his children away from him, then you've got somebody in a distressed state likely to do odd things, like try to get parental responsibility for Rhys.*

● *Dileep (1991)*

*The amount of discussion and contact women want with me varies quite a lot. It seems to have changed over the years. When I first started being a donor, the society we lived in then at the end of the GLC was much more open. In the first few cases [in the mid-1980s], I went to the women's houses, had dinner and we talked through a lot of issues. More recently I'm finding that there is much less contact. In many cases now I have no contact at all with the women. It's just a voice at the end of the phone and a third party picks up. In one or two cases there hasn't even been a third party. We've arranged that motorcycle couriers are used. This morning I was interviewed by a woman who wanted to meet me and talk through lots of issues again. A lot of the women that I'm being a donor for know somebody else that I've been a donor for, so they already have access to information about me.*

*Being a parent is something I've thought about a lot. I had thought about co-parenting in the early 1980s in one arrangement that didn't work out. Very recently one of the women who approached me about being a donor asked me if I would have minimal involvement – seeing the child occasionally. At the time she first approached me, I was involved in a relationship and my partner was very strongly opposed to that. That relationship has since broken down and I'm thinking whether I do want to go back and negotiate some contact. I haven't resolved that issue as yet and I'm spending a lot of time in counselling on it before I make a decision.*

*I haven't met any of the children. Frequently, women I'm a donor for now are friends of women I've been a donor for in the past, so I get passed on little bits of information about the existing children. Recently, the first couple I was a donor for, back in 1986, asked me to come over to talk about being a donor for the second partner in the relationship, who also wanted to have a child. I visited their home and talked this through and I saw photos of their child, who was then 4. Although I didn't meet the child, it certainly gave me a buzz to see the photo. It was really nice to know the child's name and have little bits of information about her, but I don't feel I have the right to meet that child or any of the others I've been a donor for. The child has a right to ask to see me. I've always seen it operating that way around.*

*After I was first a donor, I started thinking about what if, in fifteen years' time, the young person wants to have some contact with me, or when they are aged 3 or whatever. I've now been a donor for ten or twelve women. I think it probable that in time, maybe one or two may want to contact me, and I think I can cope with that. All of the mothers have had my consent to pass on information about me if they choose to. A few have indicated now that they do want to pass on the information. The majority say they don't. I think their decisions on that may change in the future. I've always given my consent on the basis that they may pass on information about me now or at any time in the future.*

*I'm not looking for a co-parenting relationship at the moment at all. The only way I'd see myself being involved is to meet with the child as a means of supporting the way any particular mother has chosen to bring up that child. It seems that at the age of 3 or so, a lot of children start asking questions about their fathers. From what I've read, some of the mothers then contact the donors again to see if they would be willing to meet the child. At that age, I would see myself as doing it only for the benefit of the child and not to set up ongoing contact. If a 3- or 4-year-old wants ongoing contact, I think I would primarily try and talk through with the mother or the carers in that child's life what is the best way of letting the child have a limited amount of contact with me, but without setting up regular meetings. I'm not willing to undertake that responsibility now. Once the young people get to the ages of 16 or 18 and want to have some contact with me, that's negotiable then.*

### ● Alex (1991)

*I don't want to be a parent and I don't want any involvement with the child. I think that is honest. My life doesn't allow for me to take on that responsibility – financially and everything else. I have enough problems looking after myself. I don't think there is any chance I would change.*

*I am giving sperm to Sandra who is the friend of a friend of mine. We weren't friends originally. Once I had said I was prepared to consider being a donor, I wanted to meet the woman to talk about what's involved. There are issues involved which I had never thought about before because I had never been in this situation. So we met.*

*Sandra and I decided that if we become closer friends, then my involvement with the child will be because of my friendship with her rather than just because of being the biological father. If Sandra decides she doesn't want a father around at all, that's fine. I accept that and if she decides that she wants to be open about it, then I accept that she wants to be open about it.*

*I think I am happy to be contacted by the child if the child wants to meet its father when it gets older, as long as it is quite clear from the beginning that I am not a parent. I am only a donor. There are things like that which are difficult to say yes or no to now. Sandra and I have to keep our relationship open to see if everything is all right at the time. At the moment I could say yes, that's no problem, and I don't think it would be. I used to have some fun out of the idea that I would have a photo of the child every year, and then the novelty wore off and I thought this is just some sort of a kick. It's not important for me if I don't have any involvement. But I think I would be interested in seeing the child.*

● **Mike (1991)**

*When women want me to be a donor, we meet and have a long discussion. There's a lot of trust involved and give and take. So far, it has been more or less what we both wanted. I have been prepared to go along with what they wanted.*

*I wouldn't agree to be an anonymous donor. I have a few friends who have been adopted and I know about the trouble they went through finding out about their birth parents. I would hate the mystery of not knowing where I came from and who my birth parents were. I think that children have a right to know who their father or their mother is, whether they're adopted, inseminated or whatever.*

*The women I've been donating to want their children to know who their father is, which is why I was quite happy to do it. Regardless of whether they want me to have any involvement with the child, they know who I am, so that if the child wants to get in contact with me, the mother has the knowledge and the child can make a choice. The women knew me through friends anyway so there is always a mechanism to get in contact if need be.*

*I leave the decision about the level of involvement with the child up to the woman. If she wants me to have contact with the child, I would be quite happy to get involved, but that's entirely up to her. I don't know how I would feel about being involved with the child, because it's about the future. Although I might have some fantasy about being a part-time father, I can't see into the future and nor can the women involved. If I was never to see the child, that would be fine.*

*I wouldn't mind being contacted by the children. It doesn't worry me, probably because I haven't been in that situation to know what it would be like. I sometimes fantasize that it would be lovely, like in a Hollywood movie. It could be a wonderful child that I would welcome into my home. On the other hand, it could be a grotty horrible kid coming around. I suppose it could work both ways.*

*I feel committed to carry on doing it for as long as needs be. I wouldn't feel, 'Oh I've been doing it for five months and nothing has happened. That's it.' I know that they only have a few days a month when they are fertile, and I've talked to them, and I know that it's bloody awful. It's pretty unfair when you think about it.*

*My best friend has asked me to donate for her in three years' time, but it's a bit different in that case. I've been friends with her since we were at school. It's a special friendship and has gone on for so long that I just wouldn't want anything to put it on the rocks. I would be much more cautious of doing it for her than for someone who has come along as a stranger. It might put a strain on our friendship. I don't know what she would expect from me. I'd worry that her girlfriend might feel threatened by me. If I said anything about the baby, they might think I was interfering. I don't think I will do it. I would be too scared of ruining our friendship. I'm sure she would agree, but on the other hand, she might talk me around.*

# Donor's characteristics

Potentially, a woman can choose a donor on the basis of the physical and personal characteristics she would like the man to pass on to her child. She can make a decision based on her preferences for hair colour, eye colour, race, ethnic background, religion, height and any other characteristics that matter to her. For most women, race is a bottom-line issue and they select a donor who is of the same race as themselves.

There are some women who are not concerned about the donor's features and are satisfied to find a man who is healthy, fertile and available. Others believe it is wrong to try to produce a baby with particular characteristics, fearing that the child may only be loved and wanted if certain specifications are met, and not accepted if he or she doesn't fulfil the mother's expectations. Many women want the donor to resemble themselves and/or the co-parent.

Should a woman seek out a donor from the same cultural background as herself? If she can't find one, what responsibility does she have to teach her child about the donor's cultural background? There has been much confused discussion about this issue. The majority of women are doing self-insemination because they do not want the donor actively involved as a father. They may want the child to know his identity (see the preceding section, 'Anonymous or Known?'), but in general women are raising their children according to their own culture and lifestyle and not according to the donor's. The donor is a means to having a child. I have heard of a non-Jewish woman challenged to explain how she will bring up her daughter to know and value her Jewish identity, on the grounds that the donor's mother was Jewish. The donor himself did not actively identify as Jewish. But even if the donor were a practising Jew, that would not alter the fact that his daughter is being raised by non-Jewish lesbians and he has no influence over her upbringing. Culture is not imparted through the genes but by parents who are practising and living that culture.

In practice, there are not enough men willing to be donors to have a great deal of choice. Before you start trying to find a donor, you need to think about the characteristics you ideally want in a donor and decide which are bottom-line characteristics and which are desirable but less important. If the search turns out to be long and difficult, you may well find your criteria becoming less and less strict until all that matters is that the man be healthy and fertile. This experience will reveal whether your bottom-line preferences really are as fundamental as you thought. The danger at this stage is in becoming desperate and accepting a donor whose race, ethnic background or some other feature is not what you ideally want, leaving you with a lifetime of dealing with those issues.

● *Eunice (1992)*

*Stella is white and I am black, of Afro-Caribbean descent. We talked about Stella using a black donor, but it turned out that the reasons we had for doing this fell apart when we considered that I wouldn't want a white donor for myself. In the event it was much easier for us to find white donors, but I hope this will be different when it's my turn in a couple of years. Neither of us were unduly worried about the donor's appearance. This was probably largely due to the fact that having asked several people through personal contacts and been disappointed, we had almost started to think that anyone would do. It was more frustration than despair, as we knew we'd eventually find someone, but we were also aware that finding a donor is just the beginning. I did, however, maintain certain of my principles throughout, and baldness was definitely out.*

● *Pat (1986)*

*I am black and I already had one black child. I wanted the next baby to be black. At the beginning I found it quite hard, because there weren't any black donors that I knew of. I knew about a men's group who were being donors, but there weren't any black men there. A friend and myself, who was also black, wrote to a black gay men's group at Gay's the Word [a gay bookshop] to ask for donors. They had a big meeting about it, but they said no way. They thought it was disgusting that we had the nerve to ask them to be donors.*

*I went to the British Pregnancy Advisory Service [BPAS]. There were hardly any black donors at BPAS and there were women in line for them anyway. There were three donors – one was African, one was dark West Indian and the other was pale-skinned West Indian. I didn't want a mixed-race guy. The donor of my daughter Marcy was supposed to have been the dark West Indian, but she looks mixed-race. She looks like me. Dean (my first child) is very dark. I'm not that bothered now if the baby's like me or darker. But I would have preferred Marcy to have been darker.*

*I've known women who wanted to have mixed-race babies because they think they're prettier, have nicer hair or because they want to break the norm. But how do you deal with that child when it gets older? When you're growing up being the colour I am, you're not accepted anywhere or you are accepted everywhere, depending on what the views are at the time. It gets on my nerves to think what I went through at school and as a teenager because of being mixed-race. I don't get it so much now, because I'm not that bothered, but I wish I'd been one or the other. I feel that people who want a mixed-race kid have to think about it very hard.*

*When I had Dean, I made sure that his father was black because then he'd know who he was. He wasn't going to look mixed-race. But Marcy is mixed-race like myself and I know what she's going to be saying to me when she's older about her colour. Some people are going to call her 'nigger' and other people are going to say 'You're white' or 'You're half white.'*

Even with a black parent to relate to, you're not fully black, no matter what. I call myself a black woman, but not all black people accept me. It's usually the older black people that aren't so accepting. Younger black people usually do. But you still feel you don't exactly belong. I've been told I'm too white. That's because I won't deny the white part of me – because I won't deny my mother. So you can't win.

### ● Shaheen (1992)

Although my father is from Pakistan, I was born and raised here and I don't know much about Pakistani culture. I feel very naive about it. My consciousness is white. Finding a donor at all was hard enough. I was prepared to take the first donor that came along that was healthy and willing and knew what it involved. I think I might have considered an Asian donor if it was easy to find one, but I also had to consider whether I have close friendships with black and Asian people, and actually I don't. Perhaps if my partner were Asian or black, it might have been different, but my partner was white. If I was going to have a relationship with the donor and he was going to have contact with the child, then perhaps I would consider it then. But I knew that I wanted an anonymous donor.

My brother is about the same colour as me and even though his wife is white, his daughter is very brown. I thought my son Anton would be a lot browner than he is. He is actually very white. When my partner Jackie and I were out together with Anton, a lot of people thought that Jackie was his mother and I was some aunty. Because Jackie is white and he looks white, they just put the two together, which really annoyed me.

### ● Paula (1991)

I want my daughter, Tara, to have an identity as an Asian. I never had that when I was young, because my dad, who's Asian, left when I was so young. That's why I made the decision to have an Asian donor. I thought about it a lot. I had just come back from India and I was really excited about identifying as half-Asian and identifying with Indian culture. I felt really positive about it and felt I could give a lot to a child.

I made sure she goes to an Asian childminder. I was very

*particular about that. She's been a miracle but she doesn't know I'm a lesbian. I've got a couple of Asian friends who have kids, but only one lives around here. I would like Tara to know a range of people from lots of communities. It's important to me that she should not be ghettoized. Nobody has said anything directly racist to Tara but there have been a couple of incidents and I got pissed off.*

*I'm very dubious about people who use black or Asian donors if they themselves don't have a cultural background like that of the donor. When a white friend of mine asked me if she could use the same donor [who is Asian], I said no. I met an Asian woman who was going out with a white woman and the white woman wanted to have an Asian child just like Tara – the same colour and everything, like it's some kind of a clone. She kept saying, 'Isn't she gorgeous! Isn't she lovely! Look at the colour of her skin. I want one just like that.' It's shocking what people say.*

### ● *Lesley (1986)*

*As a white woman, I would like to say something about choosing the race of the donor. I decided not to have a mixed-race donor who was offering because I didn't feel in a position to bring up a black child. I would have wanted him/her to feel part of a black community, to live closely with black adults and children. That isn't the reality of my life at present and so I felt it would be irresponsible to use a mixed-race donor. I also want my white child to grow up in a racially mixed community, to not feel he is 'normal' and everyone else is 'different', but it feels more within my powers to do that.*

### ● *Dileep (1991)*

*I made the decision that I'm prepared to be a donor for any woman who's thought through this process and has decided that she wants to have a child, so I don't need to know anything at all about her. On the race issue, I am Asian and, where I have information, only one of the women I've donated to has been Asian. There were a number that I don't know but I suspect are white, and there are lots that I know are white. I feel that that's quite positive in terms of white women now not finding it necessary any more to select out Asian donors.*

*I suppose if I weren't living in London, it might be an issue for me that there are white mothers raising half-Asian children. But with multicultural education and the way nurseries have developed, I don't think that any mixed-race child will now have problems growing up in London.*

### ● Judy (1986)

*I wanted a Jewish donor, partly because in the last few years I've got much clearer about my identity being Jewish but not defined by religion. Being Jewish for me has a lot to do with my family, and having a child is family. I wanted to have the continuity with a Jewish donor. Also being Jewish is partly about the way you look. My family came from Eastern Europe along with many Jews in England. Having a Jewish donor maximized the chances of having a child with similar 'colouring', looking Jewish like me. (This is not to be confused with selecting for 'good looks' according to the standards of the dominant culture.)*

### ● Toni (1986, 1992)

*I'm Jewish and want to raise my daughter to know she's Jewish. I strongly wanted a Jewish donor and was lucky enough not to have much trouble finding one. But if you ask me why, I don't think I can give you a satisfactory reason. It just felt more comfortable or familiar – as if he weren't a total stranger. There was some connection between us, even though I thought I would never see him again after I became pregnant. I've subsequently learned that our Jewish connection is very tenuous because he was brought up with virtually no knowledge of Jewishness. Just after Claire's birth, his identity was not very important to me, so that for a while I felt silly having made such a fuss about his Jewishness. Now that I've got to know him, I am especially glad that his family background is Jewish, and it does seem a stronger connection between us.*

## Being a donor

What motivates men who are donating sperm? What are the issues for them? When women are trying to decide whether or not to have a particular man as a donor, it is helpful to know how men might feel about it. A woman is asking a favour of someone she may hardly know. The man will give her something she wants very much but which he must be able to give without any attachment and without any real reward. She is in a vulnerable position relative to the man. He may abandon her before she conceives. He may put her at risk of HIV or other sexually transmitted diseases. He may try to claim the child at some time in the future. These are real risks and there can never be any guarantee they won't come to pass. But the more women understand what is going on in men's heads, the easier it will be to communicate with donors and to develop trust.

Luckily there are some men around for whom donating sperm is not a problem. Some are doing it as a favour to a friend and some for political reasons. It seems that for many of them, there are no long-term consequences to the act of donating. Often they are young men who are not concerned with the implications. For them, it is no big deal to be a donor. As one of the donors quoted below says, 'Although for her, it's very serious, for me it's just a toss in a jam jar.' Gay men are often the most willing donors. They are more likely to understand the difficulties lesbians and other single women face in getting pregnant, and have shown solidarity by donating sperm without complicated conditions. This suits lesbians and single women very well.

There must be some men who have found it problematic being a donor as well as many who have refused outright. It would be natural to expect that some men will later regret having been donors to a stranger and having nothing to do with their offspring. For some men, making a baby is highly emotional, even if they are not being asked to raise the child. It is reasonable to expect men who are asked to be sperm donors to have complex and sometimes confused feelings about donating their sperm. Some men have said they would not want to contribute to creating a life without taking their share of the responsibility. Others have said they would feel strange knowing half of their genes were in a person they did not know. They may worry that their anonymity will not be respected or that the mother may one day be forced to name the donor when claiming benefits, requiring him to pay child maintenance (see the section on the Child Support Act in Chapter 6, 'The Law'). This is especially the case if a man is being asked to be a donor for a woman he will never meet and whom he has no reason to trust. Girlfriends and wives may object, even if the man is willing. There are many reasons that men may give for refusing to be sperm donors. Women desperate to find donors can feel frustrated and resentful, especially if they've been searching for a long time and the man's reasons appear flimsy to them.

## ● *Alex (1991)*

*A couple of weeks after having my first HIV test, a lesbian friend of mine asked me if I would be interested in donating sperm for a friend of hers. I said I was open to the idea. I was particularly interested because I know that lesbians are having increasing difficulties getting access to sperm banks. For me donating sperm is something of a gesture of support to the lesbian community. There are so many divides between the lesbian and gay male communities. This is an opportunity to bridge gaps.*

*I have a lot of lesbian friends, which I think is quite unusual. I shared a flat with a lesbian for four years and consequently I had exposure to more lesbians than I would have normally. Also, a friend of mine is a lesbian mother. She's a wonderful example of the 'we can do it too' kind of thing. It surprises me how little gay men know of lesbians and of what things lesbians have to deal with in their lives. I believe I am quite aware of the different problems people encounter through being gay or lesbian.*

*For me this was an opportunity to do something that wasn't really any skin off my nose. I feel a bit like I am providing a service and what I am getting out of it is very little. There is an element of being used. But I have decided to be used. I have agreed. It's just a little thing.*

*There's also the area of what I can expect from being a donor. I think men have got to realize, especially in cases like mine, that I'm doing something for somebody else's benefit. Sometimes that's difficult to get used to. Not that I want fatherly involvement or any involvement with the child, but in the back of my mind, I wonder if I want something in return. Consequently I question my relationship with the woman. Do I expect something from her? Not gratitude but wanting some interest, some caring for me.*

*I know somebody who has been a donor but I haven't really talked to him about it. A lot of gay men I've spoken to have never known anybody else who's done it. To them it's a novelty. Some are quite dismissive of it. It would be nice to talk to other men who have done it. Also, it would be nice for other men who haven't done it to realize this is something that exists.*

## ● Mike (1991)

I think I'm doing it for solidarity with lesbians. I'm certainly not doing it for the kick of being a father. I have a lot of lesbian friends – more lesbian friends than gay male friends. I sympathize with them a lot. I feel I'm a good bet as a donor because, as a gay man, I would have no chance of getting custody of a child. What else is a woman supposed to do in this situation? Since I've been aware of donor insemination, I've seen adverts for donors. I think it must be awful to have to advertise in newspapers.

I've been quite fortunate with all the women I've done it for that I've met them through friends. We've just gone out for a drink and had a nice chitchat. I've been tested and I'm OK and intend to be for quite some time. I'm not going to risk my health. I have the tests to prove it and I'm available so I just think, why not? It's not that big a deal. With one woman I'm donating for, we have quite a laugh doing it. Although for her, it's very serious, for me it's just a toss in a jam jar. I can still sympathize with her and I do take it seriously. I know it's very tough for her.

It would be really nice to raise children, but being a gay person, I never thought I was likely to be a parent. I was brought up with the idea that gay people and lesbians don't have children. It has caused no problems for me. I have no great desire to find a baby somewhere. On the other hand, I've looked after my brother's kids and it's nice. I suppose in a way I do want to have children but I wouldn't force that on anyone I was donating for.

The first time that I heard about donor insemination was through a friend, who mentioned that a friend of hers was looking for donors. She told me about it, but it wasn't until about six months later that she actually asked if I would be interested in doing it for that particular woman. I had thought about it quite a lot during those six months. Initially I had been surprised. I had thought that artificial insemination, as it was known then, was something you went to a clinic for and that it was all done by doctors and nurses. I hadn't realized that it could be done so simply. When I was eventually asked whether I would consider doing it, I thought why not? What finally convinced me to do it was meeting the woman and finding out her reasons for going ahead *with donor insemination. It was quite important for me to meet her.*

*I do feel that I am very involved in donor insemination and have been quite important. In the long run I know I'm not that important, but for this part, I wasn't just a lump of sperm. I have tried to cooperate and to fit in and to be as helpful as possible. I feel that was recognized by the women I have donated for. They were so appreciative.*

● *Dileep (1991)*

*The process of donor insemination is very easy and simple and takes very little time. I've arranged to be a donor both at my home and at my office. The process just means that I ejaculate into a sterile container, which is then collected. It takes a couple of minutes each time I'm a donor. So there's no major involvement in doing this. It's not a big deal at all.*

*I first got interested in donor insemination in 1974 when a friend of mine asked me about being a donor for a lesbian woman who wanted to have a child. In those days there wasn't very much information about artificial insemination. What she had done was to ask several men to have sex with her. They had all agreed but found at the time that they couldn't do it. I thought about it and decided, without going through with it, that I also couldn't do it.*

*Then later in the 1970s I started talking in men's groups about the issues of being a donor. By that time Spare Rib was printing articles about self-insemination – how to do it and what to check for. So with that information I decided some time in the early 1980s that if ever I was asked again, I would be happy to be a donor for any woman.*

*In 1983 I completed a questionnaire for a self-insemination group. They sent me back a polite letter saying that they had put me on a register and in time women would contact me. I never heard anything more from them.*

*I responded a couple of times to adverts in City Limits in 1985. I began to think that nobody really wanted to use me as a donor because I am Asian. Eventually I got a really nice letter back from what turned out to be a Jewish couple, two women, who told me that they were very much against the blue-eyed, blond-haired concept and that they would be really happy to use an Asian donor. The first woman in that partnership conceived from first-cycle insemination. She then asked me to be a donor for a friend who also conceived in first-cycle insemination. It's all carried on from there.*

*I have continued to respond to some of the adverts in* City Limits *from time to time, but the majority of women I am a donor for know somebody else I've been a donor for before. So I tend to get passed on a lot that way.*

*The best way to get people to start thinking about being donors is to ensure that suitable articles are covered by the media – the radio or the press. The reason I've started being a donor for a clinic is that there was a programme on Radio 4 about a shortage of Asian donors. So I phoned up the clinic as a response.*

*I think there are different motivations for me in being a donor. One is certainly that I get something out of their success. The majority of women do let me know when they conceive and a bit of their excitement rubs off. Also this is just one way I feel I can contribute to a more caring, sharing society. In the 1970s a lot of people contributed to me in all sorts of ways in terms of my education on sexism and my ability to survive in society. I can't do anything at all in terms of repaying those people individually. My belief is that I should contribute where I can towards society. I don't expect anything back from these particular people I'm being a donor for, but I expect, in a society that cares, that people will contribute where they can. It's not the only way I contribute – I also serve as a management committee member in a voluntary sector project and I do volunteer driving. But this is one issue which isn't very difficult for me to undertake. There seems to be a shortage of men at the moment willing to be donors, and I don't have any problems with it on moral or ethical grounds.*

*Another reason for being a donor is something I've only recently become aware of. Some seven months ago I discovered that I'm an incest [child sexual abuse] survivor. I now know that for male survivors we tend to end up in one of three groups – abusers, victims or protectors. Protectors tend to end up in jobs working with children or people in places where they can reduce the risk of abuse. For years I've worked in crèches, in play work and in community work. Now I can recognize the 'protector role' I've been playing. It seems to me, whilst there's no guarantee that it won't occur, donor insemination children are probably much less likely to be victims of child sex abuse.*

*Initially it brought up lots of feelings for me. That mainly goes back to before I became a donor, when I talked about it in* men's groups. It brought up lots of issues about ownership, parenting, and fatherhood. I had the space then, over a period of three years, to work through a lot of my feelings with some sympathetic men. None of the rest had thought about being donors but certainly talked about it once I'd raised it in the group. I think I needed that space for myself to think through some of those issues before I could have been a donor.

● *Pierre (1992)*

My lover and I were asked by a friend if we would consider donating sperm in order that her girlfriend might become pregnant. It was explained that we would not be required to have any involvement or access to the child. I remember my lover agreeing immediately, citing the action as an act of solidarity between lesbians and gay men (though he subsequently dropped out). Whilst I agreed with this principle, for me it was a much harder decision. Looking back, I think I wondered what kind of world the child was coming into, what kind of mother Toni would turn out to be, how I would feel when the child was born knowing I could never see him or her. Having been brought up by my mother as a single parent, I had no problems with Toni's plans to do the same. I did wonder, however, what would happen if the child wanted to know about her/his biological father, and for that reason, I think I was glad the arrangement was not strictly anonymous. I figured Toni and I had friends in common, and if she needed to, she could always track me down. In the end I think I agreed because I liked Toni, respected her wish to be a lesbian and a mother and didn't think it would be that easy for her to find another Jewish donor.

The actual act of donating sperm was no big deal. On the first occasion Toni came over to our flat with a friend. We had tea and chatted. She asked us some questions about our health and family history. I guess in 1984, as a gay couple in a monogamous relationship of two years, neither of us had thought about the implications of HIV. I don't recall talking about it with Toni. Toni would call us with dates to meet at either her home or ours. We would arrive and chat for five minutes and then go into the bedroom, masturbate and ejaculate into the same jar and leave the contents by the bed. Toni would then take over. Sometimes we stayed behind and chatted. For me it was an opportunity to get to know Toni and was quite a relaxed experience.

*During the following three months, my lover and I split up and I continued to donate on my own. I felt I had made a commitment until Toni became pregnant, which she did quite quickly, and I didn't want to let her down. I have no regrets and believe it was one of the most valuable things I have done.*

Chapter two

# Screening

GIVEN that you are consciously planning to get pregnant, you have the opportunity to choose a fertile donor and to protect your baby and yourself from a number of illnesses and conditions. You can screen potential donors for HIV and other sexually transmitted diseases, as well as for inherited conditions (see the section 'How to go about screening a donor'). This is also your chance to look after your own health so that you reduce the risk to your baby (see the section 'Pre-conception care').

Unlike women who have children with their male partners, you can reject or accept a potential donor because of his fertility or health. Or you may use him as a donor but keep the information for later use. The important thing is that you have been informed and can make your own decision about using him as a donor.

There are always some risks with any pregnancy, but the chances of miscarriage or birth defects from donor insemination through clinics are no greater than normal. There is no reason to think that it will be any different for self-insemination.

Screening is necessary, but no matter how thorough your screening is of the donor or how careful you are of your health, you still cannot prevent many of the diseases or accidents that could affect you or your baby. This is no different from the situation of women trying to get pregnant by sexual intercourse.

## How to go about screening a donor

Any man who is genuine about being a donor will understand why he is being asked and will be happy to answer your questions. There are a number of ways to screen donors. If you don't want the donor to know who you are, ask a friend to do it or pretend to be the friend. One self-insemination group advertises for prospective donors. Two members of the group interview the men in public places like the Royal Festival Hall. Before the interview, they send the men a leaflet explaining what is involved in being a donor. The pair who do the interview take the information about the men back to the group, where other members of the group choose which donors they want. A sample information sheet for donors is included in this book for you to photocopy and hand out to men (Appendix B, 'Advice for Donors about Self-insemination').

The questionnaire I have drawn up (Appendix C, 'Question- naire for Donors') is meant as a guide to help you decide if you want this man to be your donor. You may find it useful to take a fuller medical history of the donor in case doctors ask for a family history if your child becomes ill. You may also want to draw up your own questionnaire or add questions of your own.

## Screening for fertility

When choosing a donor, first try to find out that he is fertile. There is no way to guarantee this but you can get a good idea from:

1. **Whether he has fathered children already**. This is the surest test of a man's fertility and worth asking him when you first interview him.

2. **Semen analysis**. Ideally, have a semen analysis done before you start inseminating. It may not be easy for the donor to get one unless it is part of an infertility investi- gation or he goes to a private clinic. Women who have access to a microscope and a counting chamber can dilute the semen and have a look. The sperm should be plenti- ful, active and normal in shape. (Specifically, there should be more than 50 million sperm per millilitre, more than 60 per cent should be motile after 1 hour, and there should be less than 30 per cent abnormally shaped sperm.)

3. **His age**. An upper age limit of 55 is recommended by the Licensing Authority set up under the Human Fertilization and Embryology Act 1990 for men donating sperm to

clinics. Pregnancy is somewhat less likely to occur with the semen of older men, though this doesn't mean that older men can't father children.

## Sexually transmitted diseases

You and your baby could be at risk if the donor has a sexually transmitted disease such as HIV, gonorrhoea, syphilis, hepatitis B (serum hepatitis), mycoplasma, chlamydia, herpes, Cytomegalovirus (CMV) and trichomonas. These diseases can be spread by semen, whether through inseminations or by sexual intercourse.

### HIV

HIV is one of the most important health issues you need to ask your donor about. It isn't enough to ask a man if he has HIV. People with HIV may not know that they are infected because they may get no signs of illness for up to thirteen years or more after infection. Others get minor or major illnesses sooner but may not be aware that these illnesses are HIV-related. You cannot tell if a man is infected by how nice he is or by the fact that he is heterosexual. You can only know that someone is infected and therefore infectious if they have a positive HIV test result. To be accepted as a donor, the man must have had a recent negative HIV test result and must be able to satisfy you that he has not been and is not involved in any current activities that would put him at risk of HIV.

A negative test result by itself is not enough to reassure you that the donor is really HIV-negative. He may be in the six-month 'window period', the time when the test could be negative even when the person is infected with HIV. A negative result means that no antibodies against HIV were found in the blood. Since it takes up to six months (and sometimes longer) to produce antibodies after infection, the test could be negative when the person does have HIV. It may also be the case that during the 'window period' before the person has developed antibodies, he may be most infectious. Because of the 'window period', no certificates of test results are going to give you a guarantee that your donor is HIV-negative.

At a donor insemination clinic, frozen sperm is used and it is possible to wait for the six-month 'window period' to pass before using the man's sperm. Clinics are required to test their donors for

HIV. When he first donates to a clinic, a donor is given an HIV test and his semen is frozen and stored until he returns six months later for another HIV test. Only if both tests are negative will his stored semen be used for inseminations. With self-insemination you are using fresh sperm. You cannot ask the man to have two tests six months apart and then only use the sperm given at the time of the first test.

Although the HIV test is essential, you still have to find out whether he could have been infected in the six months before he took the test or since. You need to ask him about any activities that put him at risk of HIV. HIV can only be spread in bodily fluids – blood, semen, or vaginal secretions – from an infected person. Bodily fluids can be passed between two uninfected people with no risk of HIV. In terms of what is important to know about your donor, you must find out if he behaves in ways which spread the virus, through any of these activities with people who may be infected:

1. **During sex.** Risky sexual activities are anal sex and vaginal intercourse without a condom and with an infected person.

2. **By sharing anything that can pierce the skin.** This means sharing drug-injecting equipment, razors or blades with people who are infected, and having tattoos, ear-piercing or acupuncture at a place that does not use disposable or resterilized needles.

3. **Through infected blood and blood products.** Blood and blood products have been screened for HIV since 1985 in the UK. In some developing countries, the blood supply for transfusion is not yet safe.

Questioning a man about activities that may put him at risk of HIV can be embarrassing, but it is the only way you can decide if you trust him. It is a peculiar position to be in. In general, donors are either complete strangers or vague acquaintances. Yet in a few meetings, you must be able to develop a sense of trust in the man. What this comes down to is that in order to know whether he is or has been at risk of HIV, you have to talk openly and honestly about sexual practices and drug use. It is not enough to ask whether he practises safe sex. Not everyone knows what this means. Hetero-sexual men may feel more uncomfortable talking freely and easily about sex than gay men. Any man may conveniently forget, or not mention without prompting, sexual encounters outside the country with strangers or prostitutes. He may have been monogamous since before AIDS was ever heard of. You still have to ask him whether his partner has always been faithful, and to have the test.

If you are satisfied that he has not been doing anything that would put him at risk of HIV in the previous six months, and he has had a negative HIV test, he can begin donating sperm. However, if he has been engaging in risky activities, he should practise safer sex or stop the risky activity for at least six months before taking the HIV test. At the end of that period, he can donate sperm if the HIV test is negative.

See Appendix A, 'Resources and Reading List', for sources of leaflets and advice on HIV and AIDS.

## HIV TESTING

Men who agree to be donors are generally willing to have the HIV test and to reassure you about their sexual practices. But not all men are prepared to take the test. They may feel completely confident that they are not at risk, or they may be frightened of a positive result. It is undoubtedly traumatic for anyone to find out that they are HIV-positive, and women need to be sensitive about this. NHS clinics offer counselling before and after the test is done, and this can help someone clarify their feelings about taking the test. However, no matter how good a man thinks his reasons are for refusing the test, it is up to you whether you want him to be your donor without a test.

HIV testing and tests for other sexually transmitted diseases are available from any NHS sexually transmitted diseases clinic (also called genito-urinary medicine or GUM clinics). They are better at safeguarding confidentiality than your GP, although GPs can also arrange for the HIV test to be done for you. Call the clinic first to see how long it takes for the results to come back. This ranges from one day to two weeks. Also check that they offer counselling before and after taking the test. To get the address of the nearest clinic or of a recommended one, you can call any of the AIDS helplines listed in Appendix A, 'Resources and Reading List'. You can also get the test done privately. If you are concerned about confidentiality, you can give a false name.

## Blood groups

It is useful but not crucial to know the blood group, both ABO and Rhesus factor, of both yourself and the donor. If you are Rhesus-negative and the donor is Rhesus-positive, the baby can be Rhesus-positive. The danger for the baby is that it could be born jaundiced as a result of antibodies against the Rhesus factor in the fetal blood produced by the mother during the pregnancy. In severe cases, the baby needs a blood transfusion. It is useful for Rhesus-negative women to know the donor's blood group so they can be monitored for this as part of their antenatal care. They will be given gamma globulin to prevent the condition developing in future pregnancies. A Rhesus-positive mother is not at risk so it doesn't matter if her donor is Rhesus-positive or Rhesus-negative.

## Genetic conditions

Through questioning the donor, you can find out if he or any of his close relatives has suffered from a genetic disorder. There are thousands of genetic conditions which could be passed on to your child by the donor or by you or by the combination of you and the donor. Most of the conditions are very rare.

Some of the conditions, such as sickle-cell anaemia, thalassaemia, cystic fibrosis and Tay-Sachs, have a simple pattern of inheritance and it is possible to calculate the odds of passing them on. If both parents are carriers of the gene, there is a one in four chance that the child will inherit the condition. As long as only one parent is a carrier, the children will not be affected though they may themselves be carriers. Carriers have no illness themselves and will not know that they are carriers unless they have been tested for the trait. If you have been tested and shown not to carry that gene, then you can decide whether to question the donor about that particular condition. You may decide that you don't want your child to have the chance of being a carrier, in which case make sure the donor is not a carrier. If you are a carrier, then only accept a donor who is not also a carrier. The tests to determine if you are a carrier are quick, simple and free blood tests, which your GP can arrange for you to have. There are organizations listed in Appendix A, 'Resources and Reading List', if you want to find out about screening for cystic fibrosis, thalassaemia, sickle-cell anaemia or Tay-Sachs.

With many inherited conditions, it is usually not possible to calculate the odds so precisely, because the patterns of inheritance are very complex and involve many genes. If any of these conditions runs in either your family or the donor's, your child could have a greater risk. A few examples: your child would have an increased risk of having a heart attack if a relative had a first attack before the age of 50. If a relative had adult-onset diabetes (the kind where the person doesn't need insulin), the child would have an increased risk of developing diabetes, especially if overweight. Hyperlipidaemia (a condition where there are abnormally high levels of fats and cholesterol in the blood) also runs in families, and someone with hyperlipidaemia has an increased risk of having a heart attack, stroke or circulation problem. Glaucoma, which can lead to blindness if untreated, is another condition which tends to run in families, as are allergies such as eczema, asthma and hayfever.

If you know that the donor has a family history of one of these conditions, you can decide to find another donor. Or you can use him and do what is necessary to prevent or monitor the condition in the child. For example, with a family history of glaucoma, the child would need an eye test every two years. If there is a family history of allergies, you can protect your baby by breastfeeding rather than bottle feeding and by reducing your baby's exposure to substances that cause allergies, such as the house-dust mite and various foods.

While many genetic disorders are inherited, some do not run in families. The chromosomes which carry the genes can be damaged by exposure to radiation, certain chemicals, alcohol or drug abuse, by age or just by chance. Men are just as vulnerable to reproductive hazards at work or in the environment as women. It is worth asking a donor if his occupation involves an increased risk of radiation or chemical exposure.

Below, three donors express their feelings on screening.

## ● *Alex (1991)*

*I had an HIV test this year but before that I had never considered donating sperm. I didn't want to take a test for that purpose alone. I wanted to take it for myself, to know about my health. Sandra, the woman I am donating for, knew that I was clear [HIV-negative]. We discussed my sex life. It was not at all embarrassing. I was clear that the restrictions that donating sperm imposed on my sex life were those that I make anyway. That means that I practise safer sex, and the risks I take for myself are the risks that she will need to take. I basically told her what my sex life involved and that if I had anal sex, then I would use a condom. But safer sex is so vague. Of course you can't get it from kissing. Indeed, shortly after I met her I started to have a relationship with somebody and we had unprotected sex. For me that was a calculated risk, because I knew that he had had an HIV test himself and I had had a test, and in the meantime both of us had had low-risk sex with previous partners. When that happened, I called Sandra and told her, because I have that responsibility to her. I felt a little bit guilty in case of what she would think.*

*I met Sandra at the end of February and we had planned to start in May. Just before we were going to do it, I had another HIV test. But the day before, I got sick with hepatitis. So that put things on the back boiler for a long time. It was just in time because otherwise I would have started to donate for her. I got sick and in August I was clear — found not to be a carrier. So I gave her my first lot in August.*

## ● Mike (1991)

*The women asked me a lot of questions about my health and what genetic diseases I had, if any. In general I thought the vetting was excellent. It was like an examination. These things have got to be asked so it's just a matter of putting up with it. It's a simple questionnaire. We had a few drinks and were laughing over it, so it wasn't actually that traumatic at all.*

*I had a sperm count done at the clinic the very first time I donated. I gave all that information to the woman I was donating to. She hadn't asked another donor to do it. He could have been infertile for all she knew. I'd hate to go through all the motions of doing it and later find out there had been no point.*

*Each time I've donated for a new woman, I've had another HIV test. Because I've been practising safe sex, I knew I had nothing to worry about. It's a hell of a lot to ask someone to take a test. I think a lot of people would rather not know. Even when I was tested and knew I was OK, I still thought, 'Oh my God, what if ...?' I know how safe I've been and the chances are a million to one that I could be HIV-positive. Even so, there's that one chance. Even after*

I'd been celibate for a year since I had a negative test, I wondered if that result could have been a mistake.

I was asked about my sexual practice and I think it's essential that women ask. You're talking about people's lives. I certainly wouldn't do anything to endanger my life, let alone anyone else's. I'm a buddy for the Terrence Higgins Trust and I just don't want to end up with AIDS. I have to look after myself. I wouldn't mislead anyone. I'm having a sexual relationship (with a man) at the moment and it's as safe as it could possibly be. The woman I'm donating to knows all about that. Basically she has to trust me. I can only be as safe as I can be.

Before I started donating for the second time, I had more thorough tests than I'd ever had before. I had tests for hepatitis, syphilis, everything. I went to a private clinic. They gave me a good deal and I thought I may as well have the works. It's so cheap now to be tested privately that I would rather go some place where you get given a cup of coffee and sit in a nice waiting room on your own. It's quicker. When I first had it done years ago, it was something like £150, but the price has really dropped. It's about £50 now, with the result the next day. I wouldn't go to an NHS clinic. I don't want to hang around for three or four weeks waiting for a result to come through. I'd sooner pay the money and know the same or the next day.

● *Dileep (1991)*

The issue of screening for HIV and sexually transmitted diseases has not come up with each woman I've been a donor for. It comes up from time to time. I've been tested about once a year for all the sexually transmitted diseases. More recently I've started to be a donor also for one of the clinics, who will regularly test me every six months as long as I continue being a donor for that clinic. If I felt I was at risk at all, I would stop being a donor. I have no intention of passing on any sexually transmitted diseases or HIV. I don't think I take part in any unsafe practices.

I feel all right when women question me about this. There have been a couple of times when women have been uncertain about asking those questions because it's a major issue for gay men. They weren't entirely happy about asking me, though I'm quite happy to answer the questions and to be tested again whenever necessary.

# Pre-conception care

When you get pregnant by donor insemination, you have to plan. There is no chance of an accidental pregnancy. While you are taking the time to organize the inseminations, you may as well take advantage of this period to prepare your body for pregnancy. Look at your lifestyle to see what you can do to increase your chance of having a healthy baby.

### Rubella

A vaccine will prevent damage to your baby by rubella (German measles). Rubella is a virus infection which can cause blindness, deafness and heart disease in the baby if the mother has the disease during her pregnancy, especially during the first three to four months. It is quite likely that you are already immune, but if you are not, you can be vaccinated. You are then advised to wait three months before trying to get pregnant, as the vaccine causes a mild version of the virus infection. Rubella vaccination does not last for ever, so even if you were vaccinated when you were a teenager, it is worth having your blood checked for immunity before you start inseminating.

### Sexually transmitted diseases

If you have any of the sexually transmitted diseases listed in the section 'How to Go About Screening a Donor', you can pass the disease on to your baby during pregnancy or at birth. The consequences can be severe for the baby, or your fertility may be affected.

### HIV

The potential risk of HIV is not only from the donor. You may be a lesbian but still be involved in some of the risky activities mentioned above. You may be raped, have sex with men for a living or have sex with men for pleasure. There have been a few cases of lesbians who have been infected with HIV through sex with other women. It may be true that lesbians as a group are at low risk of HIV, but the issue is not what group you identify with but what you do. Testing for HIV is an important decision. Get as much advice and counselling as you can, whether you ultimately have the test or not.

If you are already HIV-positive and want to get pregnant by donor insemination, you will need much more information and advice than can be given in this book. The issues facing you will be complex and difficult, made more so by hostile attitudes from the medical establishment. You will need to find non-judgemental counselling in order to help you make your own decision about the risks. Your HIV status is not the only thing to consider. You will be making a choice based on your circumstances and what you think is best for you and for your child.

Pregnancy itself does not appear to have an important effect on HIV progression, but this is based on only a few research studies. In some cases, women have progressed to HIV-related illness during pregnancy, but it's not clear whether the pregnancy was the cause of this. There is also the risk of transmitting the virus to your baby during pregnancy or childbirth. The chances of this occurring are between one in seven and rather less than one in two (between 15 per cent and 40 per cent). However, if you become infected around the time you get pregnant or during pregnancy, or if you are at a more advanced stage of HIV-related illness, the risk of transmission may be higher. A few cases of HIV transmission from a mother to an infant during breastfeeding have been reported internationally. In almost all these cases, the woman became infected near the end of pregnancy or was at an advanced stage of HIV-related illness.

Ultimately, the decision is your own and only you can make it. See Appendix A, 'Resources and Reading List', for suggestions of organizations to contact for support and counselling.

## Drugs

Certain drugs should definitely not be taken in pregnancy because they are known to cause birth defects. But it is wise to be cautious about taking any drug, especially in early pregnancy, since no drug is safe beyond all doubt. This applies to prescription drugs as well as to over-the-counter medicines, tobacco, alcohol, marijuana, cocaine and heroin. Since the fetus is susceptible from conception, avoid drugs as much as possible while you are inseminating and once you are pregnant. If you have a medical condition that requires long-term medication, you will need more specific advice from your doctor. With some disorders, such as epilepsy, the illness itself may be more of a risk to the fetus than the drug used to treat it.

## Smoking

If you smoke, you should give it up before conception. Failing that, the earlier you give up in pregnancy, the better will be the health of your baby. Smoking can make you less fertile and increases your risk of miscarriage and premature labour. Babies born to mothers who smoke are more likely to die just before or just after birth, and to be small at birth and in childhood.

## Alcohol

Drinking too much alcohol before you conceive doubles the risk of a low-birth-weight baby, who usually has more health problems than an average-weight baby. 'Too much' is more than ten units a week (one unit being equivalent to one half-pint of beer, one measure of spirits or one 4-oz glass of wine).

## Diet and nutrition

Ideally you should be eating a healthy diet that is rich in fresh foods, vitamins and minerals. In particular, your diet should be providing you with enough folic acid, calcium and iron.

Folic acid is one of the B group of vitamins, occurring naturally in a variety of foods in the form of folates. Taking extra folic acid reduces the chance of your baby being affected by a neural-tube defect such as spina bifida. It is especially important during the first 12 weeks of pregnancy. Most women are getting only about 200 micrograms of folic acid from their daily diets. The Department of Health now recommends that all women planning to get pregnant should eat an additional 400 micrograms of folic acid a day. Some foods are fortified with folic acid, such as bread and breakfast cereals (Kraft Grape Nuts, Kellogg's Special K and Kellogg's Start have particularly high levels of folic acid per serving). Check the ingredients list on the package. Other foods naturally rich in folates are dark-green vegetables (best eaten raw, steamed, stir-fried, microwaved or lightly boiled, since folate is destroyed by heat), fruit such as oranges and bananas, dairy products, Bovril, Marmite and eggs. Or you can buy folic acid supplements from chemists and health food stores. The label may say that the recommended daily amount is 300 micrograms. This is for non-pregnant adults. If you are trying to get pregnant or are already pregnant, you need a tablet with 400 micrograms (abbreviated to mcg or µg, or given as 0.4 mg).

Extra calcium is needed during pregnancy and breastfeeding. Good sources of calcium are dairy products, dark-green vegetables, fortified bread (white bread), unboiled water if the water is hard, dried apricots, sesame seeds and seed products, and fish where the bones are eaten, such as sardines.

Adequate amounts of iron are necessary for all women, but you need even more during pregnancy. Iron-rich sources are red meat, eggs, pulses, green vegetables, dried fruit, nuts and fortified cereals. If you eat offal, don't eat liver during pregnancy, because there may be high levels of vitamin A in it, which could be harmful to the developing baby.

Chapter three

# Getting Pregnant

● *Shaheen (1992)*

*The process of self-insemination and having a child was one big biology lesson for me. It taught me things I never even knew the mucus and the body was capable of doing. I was absolutely amazed. I've learned so much.*

THE aim of self-insemination is the union of egg and sperm. This section describes four steps you can take to help bring this about:

**Step 1. Fertile days** – learn to identify roughly when you are fertile but don't try too hard to pinpoint the day of ovulation.

**Step 2. Getting and keeping sperm** – get the donor to ejaculate, and keep the sperm alive and well for the next six hours while you transport it.

**Step 3. Insemination** – inseminate as often as possible (at least twice but preferably three to five times) during your fertile days.

**Step 4. Wait for two weeks.**

## Step 1: Fertile days

One or occasionally two ripe eggs are produced during a menstrual cycle in a process called ovulation. This egg is only ready and available to meet the sperm for 24 hours. However, a woman is fertile for a longer time during the cycle, ranging from two to seven

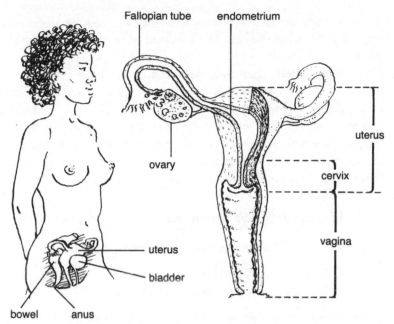

Figure 1. Where it all takes place – the reproductive organs

days (depending on the woman). The fertile days are those in which you have a chance of getting pregnant, if sperm are in your vagina. You are fertile before and at ovulation. It is these fertile days which most women can learn to identify fairly easily.

You are fertile during your fertile days due to the presence of a certain kind of mucus produced by your cervix. When sperm arrive in the woman's vagina, they are either allowed or refused entry to the uterus by the type of mucus. While the egg is ripening, the follicle (egg sac) is making the hormone oestrogen, which influences the cervix to produce thin, clear, slippery mucus. This type of mucus protects and feeds the sperm and directs them up into side pockets in the cervix. The entrance to the cervix (the os) is open. As long as this mucus is present, the sperm can survive inside the cervix, waiting for the egg to be ready. Sperm can live for three to five days as long as the 'fertile' mucus is around. Some women produce this fertile mucus for as much as six days before ovulation. As long as this mucus is present, you are fertile (unless there is some other physical or hormonal reason for infertility).

Over a period of days, the sperm are gradually released from the side pockets of the cervix to swim up through the uterus to the Fallopian tubes, where they meet the egg or eggs. Only one of the millions of sperm will bore through the jelly-like coating around the egg cell and fertilize the egg. The fertilized egg then carries on to the uterus.

Immediately after ovulation and at all other times of the menstrual cycle, your cervix produces no mucus or a thick, white, tacky mucus, and the os remains tightly shut. This type of mucus acts as a barrier to the sperm. They cannot swim through it, and in fact, they die within a few hours. No matter how active and healthy the sperm are when they arrive, they cannot get to the Fallopian tubes while this mucus is present.

## Identifying your fertile days

You can tell when you are fertile in two main ways:

1. by estimating fertile days from your cycle lengths;
2. by recognizing changes in cervical mucus.

There are also a number of secondary ways, which I will mention because they help you confirm that you have got it right and are important for women whose cycles are very irregular or whose fertile mucus is not very obvious. These are:

1. recognizing changes in the position and condition of your cervix;
2. ovulation kits;
3. ovulation pain;
4. temperature charts.

Each woman's menstrual cycles are unique. What is important here is not whether you fit into some idealized pattern but learning for yourself what is going on at any time in your cycle. This requires direct observation of your body and keeping some records, at least at first. I have included some fertility awareness charts in Appendix D for you to record whatever signs of fertility you find useful to observe.

## Estimating fertile days from your cycle lengths

Long before you start inseminations, keep a record of how long your menstrual cycles are. Count the first day of bleeding as day 1. Normal variations are 21 to 40 days. You may find that you have regular cycles with each cycle the same length, say 27 days. Or you may find that your cycles are irregular, with the lengths varying from cycle to cycle.

For most women, the day of ovulation is between 10 and 16 days *before* menstruation. The fertile days are 1 to 6 days before ovulation. Women who have regular cycles can make a rough estimation of the day of ovulation by subtracting 10–16 from the number of days in their cycle, and then estimating their fertile days by subtracting another few days from your earliest estimated ovulation day. For example, a woman with a regular 31-day cycle will have ovulated somewhere between days 15 and 21 and could have been fertile from day 10 until day 21. A woman with a regular 25-day cycle will ovulate between days 9 and 15 and could be fertile between days 4 and 15. She can then arrange inseminations to cover the fertile days. With enough inseminations (from two to five per cycle), this rough calculation is usually good enough for women with regular cycles.

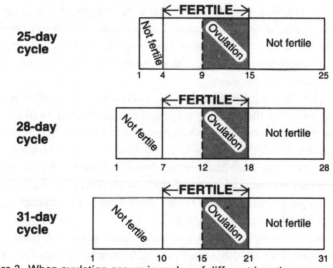

Figure 2. When ovulation occurs in cycles of different lengths

Not all women have regular cycles, though, and in any case, cycle lengths can change under the stress of trying to get pregnant. You may start out with regular cycles and find that they become irregular. Rough calculations in a very fertile woman may still be all that is necessary, even if your cycle lengths are irregular. If your cycles vary considerably from cycle to cycle, you will be much more likely to miss your fertile days. In this case, it is better to concentrate on becoming familiar with your fertile mucus.

The point about estimating your fertile days from your cycle length is that it is very rough and is based on averages for many women. You can refine your calculations by discovering just how many days before menstruation you personally ovulate (through any of the other ways mentioned below). It may be consistently 14 days. If your cycles are 31 days long, you can subtract 14 from 31 to give day 17 as the day of ovulation, and then subtract another 5 days from 17 to give your fertile days as between day 12 and day 17.

## Recognizing changes in cervical mucus

Most women notice their vaginal secretions and how they change in consistency and amount during the menstrual cycle. The secretions are made of mucus produced by the cervix plus cells sloughed off the vaginal walls. You can tell when you are fertile by becoming familiar with these changes. Identifying the changes is quite easy after a bit of practice. You simply need to get familiar with the feel of the mucus inside your vagina and to take some out on your finger to examine for stretchiness, tackiness, smell, look and even taste, if you want.

The mucus is produced in the cervix but falls to the outside and can be felt at the opening of your vagina. A convenient time to feel for mucus is after you have gone to the toilet, when you have been pushing and the mucus is more likely to have fallen to the opening. You can push the mucus down the vagina by squeezing and relaxing the muscles around the vagina. Imagine that you are trying to stop yourself urinating. This brings the mucus down where it is easier for you to reach.

Feeling and looking at the cervix itself gives you even more information. You can find your cervix by reaching deep into your vagina until you feel something smooth and firm like the tip of your nose. It is easier to do if you stand with one leg on a chair and reach in. The opening of the cervix, called the os, feels like a dimple in the cervix. You can see your cervix yourself by using a speculum, a light and a mirror (speculum and leaflets explaining its use are available from Women's Health – see Appendix A, 'Resources and Reading List').

On your non-fertile days, the cervix produces nothing or a white, tacky mucus that can look like thick icing. When you reach into your vagina and bring some out, you will find that you can't stretch it between your fingers. It feels dry. It is usually thick and sticky. It smells sharp and somewhat vinegary. The amount of mucus will vary from woman to woman and some days no mucus can be seen. The opening of the cervix (the os) is tightly closed. The vagina feels dry.

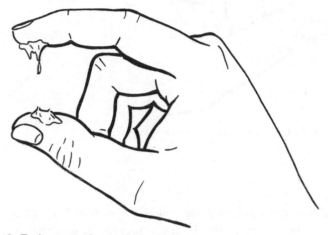

Figure 3. Tacky mucus between the fingers

On your fertile days, the cervix produces a thin, clear slippery mucus very much like raw egg white. It feels wet and slippery. If there is enough, you can pull it out of your vagina and stretch it between your fingers. Fertile mucus stretches, sometimes up to several centimetres. If you can't pull it out, you can often see the mucus on white toilet paper when you wipe yourself after going to the toilet. The smell and taste of fertile mucus is sweeter and less acidic than that of the non-fertile mucus. You can use a speculum and see the clear, transparent mucus on your cervix. With the speculum, you can also see the os open before ovulation and close afterwards.

A very clear sign of fertile mucus is the pattern the mucus forms when it is dried on a glass slide. This is called ferning and it does look like the frond of a fern. It can be seen with the naked eye, though it is best with a magnifying lens or microscope.

The only way you can tell how many days you have this fertile mucus is by looking for it yourself. Some women might produce it for two days, some for six. Again, the amount of mucus varies from woman to woman. Some women make so much that it pours out of the vagina. Others have to search to find it. The

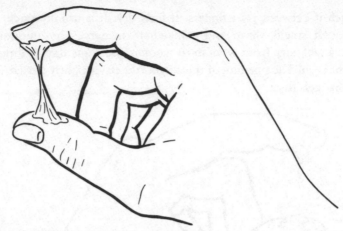

Figure 4. Fertile mucus between the fingers

amount of fertile mucus is not important, unless there is hardly any present. As long as fertile mucus is present, it is worth doing the insemination.

Your mucus observations can be disrupted by vaginal infections which produce a discharge, by some drugs and by anything which affects your menstrual cycle, such as exhaustion, stress, or travel. If you don't ovulate, you won't have any fertile mucus.

It may take several cycles before you feel confident that you can recognize the changes in your secretions and that you can tell the difference between fertile mucus and the secretions you produce when you are sexually excited. It is worth getting familiar with your cycle before you want to start trying to get pregnant.

## Recognizing changes in the position and condition of your cervix

Another way to find your fertile days is by observing the changes in the position of your cervix inside the vagina and its texture or condition. These changes come about because of the same menstrual cycle hormones that influence the production of the cervical mucus. You can add this information to your fertility awareness chart (see Appendix D).

On your fertile days, your cervix 'ripens' and is drawn up

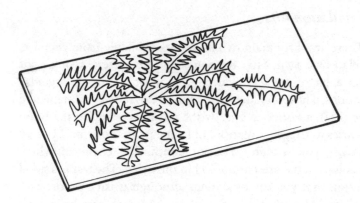

Figure 5. Ferning of fertile mucus

towards the abdomen. It feels soft, spongy or rubbery, similar to the way your lips feel to the touch. The sensation is of slipperiness because of the fertile mucus. The os opens wide. This can be felt as a dimple or a gap in the centre of the cervix and can be seen clearly using a speculum. The cervix may be harder to reach, as it moves further away from the opening of the vagina by as much as a few centimetres during the cycle.

On the days when you are not fertile, the cervix is lower and closer to the opening of the vagina and it feels firmer, more like the way the tip of your nose feels. The sensation is drier. The os is closed. If you use a speculum, you can see that the os looks like a tiny dot or a thin line.

To feel for these changes, start checking during the days when you are not fertile, as the cervix is easier to reach then. Check it once a day at the same time of day, preferably the evening, as the position of the cervix varies slightly during the day. It is generally further from the vaginal opening in the morning than in the evening. Use the same posture for checking, as posture also affects the cervix's position. You can feel your cervix by squatting or by putting one leg up on a chair and reaching in with one or two fingers. If you can't reach your cervix, try to bear down first or press lightly on your abdomen.

These signs of fertility require you to remember subtle changes in position and texture and it may take a few cycles before you feel confident about recognizing them. Not all women notice all the signs mentioned. Just record what you do notice.

## Ovulation kits

There are three main ovulation kits available from chemists – ClearPlan One Step, First Response and Discretest. Using a kit gives you a bit of advance warning, at most a day, to organize inseminations. The test is simple and fun to do. It detects luteinizing hormone (LH), a hormone sent by the pituitary gland in the brain to the ovaries to trigger ovulation. LH appears in the urine 24 to 36 hours before you ovulate. The kit contains a chemical which changes colour in the presence of LH in the urine. The test is a good confirmation that you are ovulating, although it isn't proof. You can produce LH and still not ovulate, and you can have high background levels of LH so that there are false positive results. Many women use ovulation kits together with observing their fertile signs directly, and find them very useful. You may want to use a kit for one cycle to give you confidence that you are able to recognize your fertile days.

However, it isn't essential to use a kit and they do have disadvantages, the main one being the cost. First Response costs (at the time of writing) nearly £20 for five tests plus another £12 for a three-day refill, while ClearPlan costs £20 for five tests with no refill. Another major disadvantage is that the kits focus too much on pinpointing ovulation. They can add to the stress of self-insemination and the risk that you inseminate too late.

## Ovulation pain

Although not experienced by all women, another confirmation of ovulation is pain at the time of ovulation. This may be felt as a sharp pain in the lower abdomen lasting for a few hours, or as a dull ache lasting for a day or more. In a few cases, the pain can be so severe that some women have mistaken it for appendicitis and have gone to hospital. The pain may be caused by the rupturing of the follicle (egg sac) as the egg is released, or may be something to do with the Fallopian tube.

## Temperature charts

If you keep a chart of your basal body temperature (that is, taken as soon as you wake up, after you have been asleep for at least three hours), you may notice a distinct pattern. In menstrual cycles in which you ovulate, the temperature rises very slightly (a few tenths of a degree) during the cycle and stays at this higher temperature until your next period. The rise happens a day or two *after* ovulation. By looking back on your chart, you can confirm that you have ovulated and you can tell roughly when ovulation occurred, within a two-day period. But you cannot use the chart to predict when you are going to ovulate. Most charts seem to have so many ups and downs that it is quite hard to interpret them.

The only purpose in keeping a temperature chart is to prove to yourself that you did ovulate in previous cycles and roughly when that ovulation occurred, so that you can estimate when you might ovulate in future cycles of the same length. It will not help you determine when you are going to be fertile. Some women look for a drop in temperature before the rise, but this is not the important sign: it is the rise in temperature after ovulation that is important. If you try to use temperature charts to time your inseminations, you will invariably be too late.

Emotionally, taking your temperature can be seen as a sign of commitment to getting pregnant – a statement that you have really begun the process. Equally, the act of taking your temperature every day can become oppressive. You can feel that you're not allowed to forget that you are trying to become pregnant.

See Appendix A, 'Resources and Reading List', for recommendations of books that go into more detail about temperature charts.

### Fertility awareness chart

The charts in Appendix D give you the opportunity to record all the fertile signs you have been observing. Check each of the signs once a day for two or three cycles and you should have a good idea when you are fertile.

# Step 2: Getting and keeping sperm

The man's contribution to fertilization is a small quantity of fluid called semen. Semen is easily collected by asking the man to masturbate and ejaculate into a clean jar, preferably plastic or porcelain. Plastic food containers, particularly yoghurt pots, are ideal. The jar doesn't have to be sterile but should be well washed and rinsed of all traces of detergent. Metal and styrofoam may harm the sperm. The use of a condom is not a good idea, especially not one impregnated with spermicide.

The amount of semen should be somewhere between 2 and 6 millilitres (ml) – 1 ml is about one-quarter of a teaspoon. If there is less than 1 ml, the man probably has not ejaculated properly. If you can, ask him to do it again.

Semen should be milky-white or grey-white with a characteristic odour. If it is greeny or browny coloured and/or has an extremely unpleasant pungent odour, it is likely that the man has an infection or is bleeding somewhere in his genito-urinary tract. It may still be fertile but should not be used. Semen which is very clear (like saliva) usually contains very low numbers of sperm and shouldn't be relied on for self-insemination.

In each millilitre of fertile semen, there are 50 to 100 million sperm, more than enough for fertilization. The number of sperm is not as important as their shape and motility (their speed and the way they move), which you can see under a microscope. Donors should not be advised to abstain before each insemination. It's a myth that abstaining from ejaculation for two or three days will improve the sperm count or strengthen the sperm in any way. Sexual activity in general increases sperm production. The man should have ejaculated three to four days before the first insemination. If he has not ejaculated for the previous ten days, his sperm count goes down. The use of broad-spectrum antibiotics in the seventy days before the inseminations may also decrease the man's sperm count.

Immediately after ejaculation, the semen clots, but within twenty minutes, it liquefies. It is then easier to suck it up into a syringe.

Sperm are more robust than we have been led to believe. Outside the body, sperm will live for many hours in seminal fluid if there is enough fluid to prevent drying out. In vitro fertilization (IVF) is a technique in which a woman's egg is fertilized by mixing it with sperm outside the body in a Petri dish. In IVF laboratories, sperm are kept in a simple salt solution for six to eight hours before they are mixed with the eggs, and those not used for inseminating eggs swim about for days at room temperature. Sperm can be kept for even longer, three to five days, in a culture medium and still bring about successful IVF.

Women doing self-insemination can prolong the life of the sperm and avoid anxiety about the length of time between ejaculation and insemination. Sperm live longer (at least six hours and probably more) if they are not allowed to dry out and if they have little contact with air. There are two simple measures which help:

1. Put the semen in a tall, thin pot rather than a short, wide one. Or suck it up into the syringe as soon as it has liquefied, secure the plunger and wrap the syringe in clingfilm.

2. Dilute the semen with a salt solution. You can buy a 20-ml sachet of Normasol from any chemist. This has the right concentration of sodium chloride. Add a couple of pinches of pure sodium bicarbonate (**not** baking powder) and mix one part semen to one part solution. Don't dilute the semen too much. Never mix semen with water, as the sperm will explode.

You can carry the semen around at room temperature or body temperature but certainly not any warmer. It is safer to keep it too cool rather than too hot. You can keep the jar next to your skin while in transit, but this is not an obligatory part of the process. Heating the sperm by placing the jar in front of a fire or in direct sunlight will kill them.

Some women mix the semen from more than one man at each insemination in order to make it more difficult to identify the father. There is recent evidence that this isn't a very good idea, as the sperm may block each other. With the availability of genetic fingerprinting tests, it would still be possible to conclude which donor was the biological father if the man were determined to pursue this.

## Step 3: Insemination

Any implement which moves the semen from the jar into the vagina will do. A 5-ml or 10-ml plastic needleless syringe is the most convenient but, if necessary, even a spoon will do the job. Plastic syringes can be ordered from Women's Health (see Appendix A, 'Resources and Reading List'). Many chemists sell syringes but want to be reassured that they are not going to be used for injecting drugs. One woman allayed the chemist's suspicions with a story about using the syringe to administer medicine to her cat. Try saying that you need it to water seedlings or to irrigate a wound. You only need one syringe as it can be reused each time. Wash it and rinse it well but do not boil it. You can also use eye-droppers, wide plastic drinking straws with a teat, cooking syringes, or syringes from paint shops for mixing paint. Practise sucking up milk with the syringe before you do your inseminations so you don't risk losing any of the semen on the day.

It is easiest to wait until the semen liquefies before you inseminate. Try to put the semen as close to your cervix as possible. This gives the sperm a head start and saves them from a long, exhausting swim through the hostile environment of the vagina. Near the cervix, the fertile mucus protects and directs them through the os.

There are several ways to keep the semen in your vagina long enough for most of the sperm to end up in the right place. The simplest is to lie down for 15 to 30 minutes with your buttocks raised – a pillow will do. If your uterus is in the most common position, that is, tilted forward towards your front or lying straight, it is best to lie on your back. But if your uterus is tilted backwards, you may be more successful lying on your stomach. You only know the position of your uterus after a pelvic examination by an experienced person. The semen will drip out when you eventually stand up, but enough of the sperm will stay inside. Thin sanitary pads are handy for catching leaks.

A diaphragm or a cervical cap (a small thimble-shaped contraceptive device which fits by suction over the cervix) will hold the semen directly against the cervix. If using the cap, the semen is placed in the cap before it's put in the vagina. Cervical caps should be available from family planning clinics but they may be difficult to get. If you use a diaphragm or cap, you do not need to lie down after the insemination.

## How many inseminations?

It is, of course, possible to conceive after only one insemination. However, you will maximize your chances of getting pregnant by doing at least two and preferably three to five inseminations in each cycle. (See Chapter 7, 'When SI Isn't Working'.)

The more often you do the inseminations within the fertile part of the cycle, the more quickly you will become pregnant.

## Arrangements to get the semen

The ease of collecting the sperm and doing the insemination is often cancelled out by the awkwardness of the arrangements to get the sperm to the woman while she is fertile and within two hours of ejaculation. It can go smoothly, with everything working out as planned. The simpler the arrangements, the more likely this is to happen. All too often, however, the arrangements end up particularly complicated and stressful. This is especially so where either the woman or the donor prefers to remain anonymous. They must use intermediaries to pass the semen and must co-ordinate the transfer carefully to make sure the minimum of time passes between ejaculation and insemination. Where both want to be anonymous, each appoints an intermediary to act on their behalf. In this case, not only must the woman and the donor be prepared to drop everything else during her fertile days but both intermediaries must make themselves available at short notice. Everyone must be flexible, available and easily contactable to carry these kinds of arrangement off smoothly. If the woman doesn't conceive by the first or second month, her disappointment and anxiety can be compounded by the unpleasantness of having to ask strangers for a big favour. Sometimes donors and friends drop out after several months, leaving the woman to make new arrangements.

Where the donor and the woman agree to meet, the arrangements are usually less complicated. A woman may have the donor come to her home, she may go to his home or they may both meet at someone else's. Some donors will meet the woman but insist that she be using other donors at the same time, in an effort to keep the father's identity unclear. In practice, donors are hard to find and women are put in the position of either saying they are using more than they are or making three times as many arrangements.

# Step 4: Wait for two weeks

After you've done your first round of inseminations, there's nothing more you can do until your period is due. Even if you've done everything you could to arrange a fruitful meeting between your egg and his sperm, the result is still up to chance.

How will you know whether it has worked? You will almost certainly be thinking about it constantly and watching your body for the slightest changes. There are many signs of pregnancy. Not all women experience them and none by itself is a sure sign of pregnancy. Some women notice changes a week to ten days after conception. Others feel nothing different until weeks after they have missed a period. Common signs are breast swelling and tenderness, nausea, more frequent urination, tiredness, more vaginal secretions and constipation. A missed period is somewhat more conclusive, especially if you were able to pinpoint ovulation fairly accurately. On the other hand, a period doesn't necessarily mean that you are not pregnant. Some women have a scanty bleed when the fertilized egg implants into the uterine wall. If you have been recording your basal body temperature and it is still high 20 to 22 days after the temperature rise following ovulation, you can be fairly sure that an egg has been fertilized.

There are several home pregnancy testing kits available from chemists. Clearblue, Predictor, Discover Today, Boots Home Pregnancy Test and First Response are the main ones on the market. All pick up the hormone HCG (human chorionic gonadotrophin) produced by the placenta, which comes out in your urine or blood. The kits cost between £8 and £11 and will be accurate as early as one day after your period should have started. It's best to buy a double kit so you can do a second test if you do the first one too early. The test done through a doctor is reliable 41 days after your last menstrual period. It has the advantage of costing nothing and will confirm what you may already know by this time.

## ● *Eunice (1992)*

*Having read so much about pinpointing the fertile period – temperature charts, mucus tests, chemical thingies in test tubes – ClearPlan launched their ovulation detection kit just around the time that we (my partner Stella and I) were due to start inseminating. We had already had a run-up period using the less expensive methods and thought that we had cracked it, but the idea of just weeing on a stick and looking for a colour change seemed so much easier. It worked well for us, although other people haven't found them so useful. They are also expensive and I remember going to as many branches as possible of a well-known chemist to collect money-off vouchers which were part of the launch promotion. We were also lucky with cooperative donors. We would give approximate dates from one month to the next and then confirm nearer the time. I also think that the fact that this tended to fall towards the end of the week and usually at weekends made arrangements easier.*

*It took eighteen months for Stella to get pregnant and I think that we always did something slightly different, each time thinking that we must have found the reason why it hadn't worked the time before. Initially friends did collections for us and Stella would inseminate at home, but we ended up collecting ourselves and just doing it in the back of the car. This was much easier than it sounds and actually lightened things up, as we ended up laughing at the ridiculous traffic situations we got into. This was the method that worked in the end. It could just be that our time had come and it would have worked anyway – who knows?*

## ● Toni (1986)

*My first attempts were through the friend of a friend who had persuaded a men's group to donate sperm. These men were heterosexual and very anxious that I never lay eyes on them and that their girlfriends never lay eyes on me. This is what happened the first month. After telling my friend my fertile dates, she called her friend [the intermediary] and relayed this information. The intermediary contacted three men from the men's group with the dates. She or they had insisted that two men must donate for each insemination. The argument I was given was that the second is a back-up in case the first has nerves and can't get it up. The intermediary called my friend and gave her one date for the insemination out of the three I needed. I felt cheated but could do nothing about it.*

*On the big day, my friend drove me to the intermediary's house and parked around the corner while she went in to collect the first man's semen. He had arrived ten minutes earlier with his semen already in a jar – how long ago that had happened I had no idea. Instead of going home to do the insemination, the intermediary jumped into the car and directed us halfway across London to get the second man's semen, all the while cursing me for being in the car, as even she wasn't supposed to see me. She stormed out to his house, coming out twenty minutes later, looking conspiratorial. We drove her home, another twenty minutes, and then tore across London at 80 m.p.h. to do the insemination at home. All the while,*

*I was alternating between terror at losing my life in a car crash, and terror at losing my sperm to a premature death with every minute that passed. At home I was a nervous wreck and spent the next hour lying comatose without even the energy to summon welcoming thoughts about the sperm.*

*That happened three months running. The last time, I arrived late and found the intermediary had gone out, leaving the jar of semen sitting on a stool a foot away from a blazing fire. Needless to say, the sperm were cooked, and I didn't use it.*

*I asked around for another donor. My new lover knew of a gay couple who fortunately agreed to be donors but not fathers. After the last experience, I didn't care any more whether the donor was anonymous. All that mattered to me was that the semen be absolutely fresh – no more than minutes old. My lover and I went to their house and chatted for a while. They both ejaculated into the same jar and left it by the bed. As soon as they came out, I went straight in and did the insemination. I never got used to the semen but I became more relaxed during the three months it took to get pregnant and stay pregnant.*

● *Cathy and Jean (1986)*

## Jean

Cathy (my lover) made a contact through work for her self-insemination – getting some sperm from a gay donor through two other lesbians who were also lesbian mothers. It was quite an exciting adventure. The sperm was handed through the door in a jar. The two women had the syringes bubbling away on the stove. We'd all have a chat. I remember the first time while Cathy was lying on the couch with a glass of wine, one of them said, 'Now, make sure you squirt it in, fast. Really squirt it in. You want to get it right up by the cervix.' It was great fun really. I did the inseminations. [Cathy conceived that time and had a baby girl in 1984.]

### Cathy (about Jean's attempts at self-insemination)

Jean thought she was going to get pregnant really easily. She thought she had regular periods. So she didn't think she had to do much work around finding out when she ovulated.

## Jean

Every now and again I don't ovulate and have a short cycle. I've always considered myself as having regular periods, but then when I look back on them, they're not at all. They range between 21 and 28 days. They probably were regular until a few years ago. And then they started to change. I have a very accurate record of eight or nine months of periods, with mucus changes written down in my diary. And I can predict, usually, when I ovulate. I think I should inseminate at the first sign of mucus, at optimum mucus and again after the mucus is starting to disappear. I haven't been able to do that in all the time I've been trying because of difficulties with getting the sperm.

One donor didn't live particularly close – a 15-minute fast car ride away. You're driving back with the sperm between your legs, changing gear and once when I got back with it, Cathy had melted the syringe! That was just the pits! I wanted to throw the sperm on the kitchen wall, and Cathy just said, 'Oh well, you've got it now. Come on, we'll use this plastic spoon.' I was really cross and angry and upset and tired, from a stressful day at work. That on top of it.

I think that only one month did I inseminate twice. Mostly we could only manage once. Nobody else was involved except me and Cathy. I started going to pick up the sperm myself and bringing it home and inseminating. It was just miserable.

## Cathy

It's always better to get someone else to pick up the sperm, not to do it yourself. And preferably not your partner either. It's better for you to relax. You don't want direct contact with the donor at that stressful time. It isn't that you don't want to know the bloke, it's just difficult to ask. You are dependent on him for something extremely important to you, and which he can be very flippant about. You just want to avoid contact so as to avoid getting hurt and feeling put down.

I think Jean felt very upset but didn't know quite what was wrong for a few months. That was difficult. It wasn't for a few months that she said that she hated doing it and had this horrible feeling about it. It was much better when she could admit that he was just the wrong donor. The whole circumstances were wrong. It *didn't feel right. Except that in her desperation to get pregnant, she tended to push herself. It's not worth pushing yourself on. You've got to stop if it's not right. I don't think there was much chance of Jean getting pregnant in those circumstances somehow.*

## Jean (1987)

*[Now a mother after trying a donor found through advertising.] The fact that my donor could come to the house made life a hundred times easier. The time I got pregnant, Cathy and the baby had popped out shopping and there was only me and another woman in the house. I answered the door to him and offered him a drink, but he was in a hurry, so he went straight upstairs to my room, where a clean jam jar was waiting. In a very short time he was finished and I saw him out. I rushed up to inseminate. I had everything ready – a sterile syringe, towel to lie on and book to read. For ages I'd asked Cathy to help by putting the semen into my vagina, but I'd recently realized that I wasn't entirely happy with this, as it made me tense. I was much happier doing everything myself, as I did that morning. The house was very quiet and I lay still and relaxed for nearly an hour, fantasizing about rocking my baby in my arms. I needed that time on my own to daydream about the future.*

## ● Bronwen (1986)

*I had so much fun arranging my late-night self-insemination assignations. I would get my room all ready so that when I got into bed I wouldn't have to get up again all night to fetch a book or a glass of water. The whole situation appealed to my sense of farce, and often I would laugh out loud at my fumbling attempts not to spill the jar of sperm during my attempts to draw it up into the syringe. The first month I tried I had bought a 10-ml syringe – very optimistic. Most of the sperm remained in the nozzle. And so the second month I went to the other extreme with a 1-ml one, and that time was filling it time and time again, most anxious not to get air bubbles in as I had heard that was a bad idea. Well, bad idea or not, it worked fine and 39 weeks later I stood up and gave birth to Rhys in triumph.*

### ● *Mike (1991)*

*I don't mind being flexible because I know that pinpointing the actual day of ovulation causes a lot of trauma. I try to fit in with what times are best for the woman I'm donating to. We come to an arrangement about what time of the day it's going to be.*

*One woman I donated to used to come around to my house. I would go into the bedroom and she would watch television. I was able to cope OK with that. Another woman arranges for a friend to pick it up. The first time I did it for her, I had five lesbians outside in the car beeping the horn and I just could not get aroused. It was dreadful. There's nothing worse than someone calling and saying we'll be there in ten minutes' time. It made me think that I was impotent. Since then we've come to a great arrangement with a friend who lives around the corner. I do it and when I'm ready I ring the friend up who comes to get it. I feel much more in control.*

### ● *Dileep (1991)*

*I've now been a donor for fifteen women. As long as women continue to conceive, it makes sense for me to continue to be a donor. It seems to go in phases where several women contact me at one time and then there's months of not being a donor at all. My experience has been that the first seven were successful in the first and second cycle of insemination. Then that was followed by one woman who failed to conceive for five months, started to use an ovulation kit and conceived in the first month of using the kit, but lost the pregnancy at twelve weeks. At the beginning of this year, she started again and conceived in her first cycle. There were two women who failed to conceive using me for six months. They stopped and wrote to say how disappointed they were and couldn't understand why they hadn't conceived. One had been pregnant previously. It is very disappointing. Then at the beginning of this year there were two more successes – one first cycle, one second cycle. Now I'm a donor for one woman who's at her fifth cycle of inseminations and two who have got to second cycle.*

*Most women go for two inseminations per cycle. In a few cases, I've been asked to inseminate three times for a cycle. That seldom causes any problems for me but occasionally I'm not available for a particular insemination. I've always worked on the basis that it's down to being able to fit in with my time, and so far I haven't really had any difficulty with that, so if somebody wanted me to be a donor three or four times in a cycle, I don't really see that that would pose any more problems for me than the present arrangement. It's only if arrangements can't be made for picking up at times that are mutually convenient.*

Chapter four

# Singles and Couples

## *Doing it on your own*

WOMEN doing self-insemination without a partner are
making a conscious decision to go it alone. This may be a positive
choice or it may be a second-best option. But this chapter is for all
women, even those starting off in a co-parenting partnership. The
reality is that couples do split up and people do die and become
seriously ill. Any mother can become a single parent through circumstances outside her control.

It's not always possible to have such control over your life
that all your plans work out the way you want them to. You may
prefer to have a partner first but feel you cannot afford to wait
while your fertile years slip away. Or you may find yourself with
such a strong desire for a child that a partner can wait but the desire
cannot. It may feel like the only way you can be a mother, even
though you would rather not be on your own. Whatever the reason,
choosing to be a single parent for many women is a response to less
than ideal circumstances. It may be easy to come to terms with this
reality, or it may be very painful.

There are women who would rather parent on their own
than in a couple. You may be someone who doesn't see coupledom
as part of your life plan. Although there is intense pressure from
both heterosexual and lesbian society to be part of a couple, in fact
not everyone sees it as a necessary way to live their life. There are
advantages in being the only one who makes all the decisions and
does all the work. It cuts out the arguing with an uncooperative or
unreliable mate. There are no unrealized expectations, no one else
to blame if things go wrong. There is no confusion about who is
responsible for what, no jealousy between partner and child. Given

the rate of relationship breakdown, you may prefer to come to terms with it from the beginning rather than have it thrust upon you.

## Realities of being a single mother

Women who choose to become single mothers know that they are taking on full responsibility for another person. Single parenting is undoubtedly a major responsibility in a society which is fundamentally unsupportive of mothers. Most lesbians do not have the active support of extended families or communities and certainly not of society. The lesbian community is no more oriented towards children and mothers than society as a whole. It is important to recognize the extent of the responsibility a single mother has to carry. You will be responsible for earning the money you need, organizing childcare while you work and socialize, maintaining your household, looking after the emotional and physical needs of yourself and your child, and making endless decisions for your child.

A recurring feature in the life of single mothers is exhaustion and lack of time, especially when the children are very young. When a mother is exhausted, she tends to be irritable, miserable and prone to illness. You cannot enjoy your children when you are tired and sick. You can feel that you are juggling a set of impossible demands, with no chance of a rest.

Another common feature of single parenting is isolation and loneliness. The company of babies and small children, however much you love them, is not sustaining for long periods of time. Adult company is a basic need and one to be respected, as is time alone out of the house away from children.

Building up a support network is an essential part of single parenting and one that most single mothers become quite good at. It can even be fun. Parenting is one thing that cannot be done on your own in isolation from other people. If you think you are self-sufficient and capable before you get pregnant, you will soon learn that you definitely need other people. You need it not only for your own mental health but for the sake of the child. The demands of single parenting are so great that most single mothers become aware of the importance of prioritizing their needs before they go under. You can find support from your family and friends and from other single mothers. You won't get far if you wait for it to come to you. Occasionally, people will offer, but as a general rule a single mother has to put considerable energy into organizing the support she needs. This may be physically and emotionally exhausting but may also be rewarding and fun. Many women find they make lifelong friendships through the support networks they create as single mothers.

## In the lesbian community

Being a mother is something that more lesbians are choosing to do, but there is still little acceptance of mothering in the wider lesbian community. This is changing gradually as more lesbians are visible about their parenting activities. Many mothers find that their circle of friends changes to include only lesbian mothers or only other mothers. Lesbians who have chosen not to parent may be critical or threatened by lesbians who consciously choose to do so, especially by those who are doing it alone and appear to need more support. They may feel or even say that if you had a child on your own, that's your choice and you should live with it. This attitude is a reflection of society's view that children are a commodity belonging to the parents and not a responsibility of society. They may phrase it in ideological terms about lesbians taking their energy away from other women, but it comes down to the same thing. It may even feed into your own doubts and make it that much harder to reach out for help.

Where there is acceptance of lesbians as mothers in the lesbian community, it may be only if you fit into the stereotype of the lesbian family, which is of one or two children living with their two mothers who are living together and in a sexual relationship with each other. While this family type is one valid lifestyle among many, it is not the ideal we are all aiming for. What is unique about lesbian families is not that our children have two mummies instead of a mummy and a daddy but that we are lesbians raising children without men as fathers. Without this recognition, lesbian single mothers become invisible in the lesbian community.

One of the issues for single lesbian mothers is about visibility as a lesbian. Other lesbians may assume that you are heterosexual or accuse you of passing just because you are single. The invisibility that single lesbian mothers experience is a consequence of the prevailing judgement that women should be part of a couple. This of course applies equally to heterosexual and bisexual single mothers. You do not cease to be a lesbian if you are not currently sexually active or if you do not have a live-in lover. It may be hard enough to be single without losing your identity as a lesbian in the process. Another side of the visibility issue is that all lesbian mothers, whether single or in a couple, can and do decide to pass as single heterosexual mothers in some circumstances. A lesbian who constantly passes as heterosexual will be giving very confusing messages to her children and doing damage to her own self-esteem. But there is no obligation on lesbians to be out in every situation. Every mother must make her own decision about what is appropriate or what she can deal with.

Finding support from the lesbian community may or may not be successful, but it should be possible from other lesbian mothers. There are lesbian and children groups which provide social and moral support for both the mothers and the children. Where these exist, there is a way to counter some of the isolation a single mother experiences. It takes energy and time to clarify what everyone's expectations are of such a group, but if it works out, it can be very important to single mothers. Less formal support and friendship networks with other lesbian mothers are also important. As a single mother, you may find that your needs for reciprocal childcare arrangements and visiting are greater than those for mothers in couples. Women raising children in couples often try to satisfy all their needs within their nuclear family setup. They may need as much time away from their children as the single mother does, but often do not recognize this. This can be very frustrating for the single mother and tends to leave her more isolated and lonely.

There is much that the single lesbian mother has in common with single heterosexual mothers. Self-help groups for single parents can be a good source of support. But the differences are not trivial. Besides their possible homophobia, the fact that you have done self-insemination and chosen to get pregnant by yourself sets you apart from women who have been abandoned by men and feel bitter about being on their own. They may be coming together to commiserate with each other on the awful situation they have been left in. They may not be enthusiastic about your positive decision to be a single parent. On the other hand, the experience may be very rewarding.

## Starting new relationships

The state of being single or in a couple is rarely permanent. Relationships split up and new ones start. Motherhood and sexuality are not irreconcilable. Meeting someone may be harder for single mothers, either because of tiredness or because babysitters won't stay past 10 p.m. If you do find a lover, there is a host of issues that can complicate the new relationship.

There is inevitably less spontaneity about being sexual when there are children around. This can be disappointing and frustrating for both you and your lover. You have to organize and structure your time so that both your children's needs and your sexual needs are met. There is bound to be lover–child jealousy, with mothers feeling torn between the two, even when both lovers are mothers. A single mother's primary commitment is to her child, and this may be hard for a non-mother lover to accept. Adults have the right to privacy and to prioritize sexual and intimate relationships.

Although jealousy is inevitable, many children of single mothers are also or eventually pleased that their mothers are happier. An intense one-to-one mother–child relationship can be a burden on a child, especially if the mother is unhappy. Children do feel responsible for their parents and may even be relieved that there is someone else around who can share that responsibility. The dynamics of the mother's relationship to her child will change when there is a lover. She may find herself protecting her child from being left out or from a lover who is jealous of the child or not used to children. Equally, the relationship of the lover to the child is something that can be discussed but not forced. You may or may not want your lover to become a co-parent, but if you do, your children may not accept another mother. A lover has no clear status or authority over your children.

It may be much harder to choose to have more than one child if you are on your own. Some women are not put off and will have a second or third child without a partner, but many women who would like several children reluctantly decide that one is enough. This can cause a lot of sadness.

● *Sheila (1992)*

*I chose to do it alone. I know lots of women who want a baby but who first of all want a partner. It was never like that for me. This was my own life decision, something that I was choosing for myself. Being part of a couple with somebody has never been a major goal in my life. If it happens, OK, and at times I do feel more drawn to it than at others. But it's not a part of my basic life plan. Therefore the decision to have a child wasn't made in that context. It was more that I was choosing whether or not I wanted to do it for myself. It didn't feel like a second-best solution.*

*When I first decided to get pregnant, I was lovers with a woman named Liz but we didn't see ourselves as a couple. We had no intention of being together for years and years. That wasn't our philosophy. We were lovers for about four years but we didn't live together until she decided to move to the town where I was living and spent ages looking for somewhere to live. She ended up living in my flat but we still tried to maintain separate lives. When I made the decision to get pregnant, Liz was against the idea. She moved out and we stopped being lovers shortly after Tim was born.*

*I feel happy that the decision to do it alone was right for me. It was the best thing I ever did, the best life choice I ever made. In terms of my relationship with Tim, I think it's brilliant. That side of it is easy. But I do think it is hard doing it on your own, especially the practical details. It's hard having no money when you're the only one there to pay all the bills, and living with other women has its own hassles. I've tried both and I'm happier living on my own with Tim.*

*I suppose a lot of single women think that eventually they will meet someone, but I've never had that expectation. It is difficult not having support for me that's automatically built into our living situation. I have had to learn to be my own strength, to cope alone with things. There's good and bad in that because it makes me more isolated, yet at the same time I have learned to get emotional support from a number of people rather than from one.*

*I strongly value those support networks and close friendships with other people. It makes me sad when women in couples let those friendships drop. It's not just important for the mothers but for the children too. I can't quite imagine how the children would cope if they thought they were the only ones with a lesbian mother. I go to some lengths to make sure that they have those relationships. When I was young, I had lots of cousins and we went on outings, birthdays and parties together. I suppose that the way I grew up influences what I want now. I always had the idea that I would make that for myself and choose my own family.*

*I used to say to my friends that I wanted our children to be like cousins to each other. I feel really happy that we've managed to do that. Most of my closest friends are other lesbian families. Some of them were in the original self-insemination group with me, and those children are 12 or 13. We are also close to other younger children and their lesbian mothers and we spend lots of holidays and weekends together. This loose network – my 'chosen family' – is an important part of my life and Tim's. It makes me feel really pleased and proud of what we have done and how we have managed to struggle with those relationships. They haven't always been easy. It is really like my mum and her sisters. You have rows but you come through them and stick with it. That's a commitment I've made for the children and for me and my friends.*

*Since Tim was born, I have had long periods of not having a lover. In the past I worried about whether it would be difficult when I do have a lover. What happens in reality is that Tim has always been very welcoming to the lover. It amazes me how really easy and nice Tim always is about it. He's so warm and encouraging to them. I think it's because he thinks I'm happier with a lover and that he sees it as a bit more fun than our boring old life with just the two of us. I've never lived with a lover, so it doesn't ever get to be ordinary. We did go through some quite difficult times with the first lover I had in his life. He was 6 when I got involved with her. He sometimes felt left out, and sometimes I felt quite torn between my needs and his needs. One thing I learned from that first relationship is that I expected her to love him as much as I loved him or as much as she loved me. I felt critical of her for not loving him enough, and it took me a long time to realize that that was an unreasonable expectation. It took somebody else who was lovers with a mother to say to me, 'Of course the thing is that the mother always thinks you are going to love their child as much as them.' I had a flash of realization of how it felt to be in the other position. Years later I had a relationship with a mother and I think there's quite a difference between having lovers with children and those without. The dynamic is different. Having any kind of lover requires quite an adjustment. It is a shift in the balance of relationships. Luckily Tim is into talking about it.*

*A lot of people have the idea that children can only cope with long-term relationships. I don't agree with that. I think children can and do cope. Anyway, what can you do about it? It's life, isn't it? There are all sorts of situations where you have close friends for short periods. Children do that too. My attitude with lovers is to let it develop into a close friendship if it is going to. I've never kept a lover away from Tim. I make sure I do have time with lovers when he's not there, but not only. I couldn't imagine just having a lover who wasn't involved with him as well. I think it's very nice for them to develop a close relationship, but if it ends, then it ends.*

*An important person in our family is my close friend Anna. She was my first lesbian lover and we went on being friends after we were no longer lovers. Although she wasn't welcoming of my pregnancy, she quickly became involved with Tim when he was very tiny. The three of us have seen her as a kind of second mother, though not perhaps as an equal parent. If I die, Tim would live with her. She's been very involved in his life. I think it's really important for him to have other adults whom he is close to apart from me. So from that angle, I am committed to making sure that their relationship goes on. If he goes to her for a weekend, I will do what needs to be done to organize it and get him there. We've had some conflicts. When I moved out of London, she felt really angry and powerless about it, saying that I was taking him away from her. In fact, we've made it so that he spends whole weekends with her and holidays. Like any other relationship, there have been times when I've felt like saying we should forget it and let go of it. But I'm strongly motivated to keep on with it. That's because I believe that it's right even though I feel angry with her about some choices she's made in her life. I just have to respect their relationship and let them get on with it.*

*Because a single parent needs other people to be with their children, sometimes those relationships can develop much more than if the mother had a partner. I needed holidays alone or with my lover and Tim would go off with someone else or spend time with other people. It's a normal part of his life to do that. There wouldn't have been as much space for Anna if I had had a partner or if Tim had had another involved parent. I've seen it happen with children I know, where there's so much adult input at home that there's no need for any other grown-ups outside the immediate family. So the children don't learn to be flexible. That's something Tim has learned − to be really flexible, to make the best of any situation, to really enjoy different experiences. I've seen some children who find that very difficult, partly because they're not used to it. I'm happy that he has had that.*

● *Toni (1992)*

*I chose to get pregnant on my own. I don't regret the decision because I love my daughter Claire so much, despite all the pain of parenting, and because I don't see what else I could have done.*

*Ideally I wanted to have a partner to share this activity with, but I had little confidence in my ability to form a secure, long-term relationship. I was in a rocky relationship with a woman at the time I made the decision, but I never saw her as having any long-term part in my plans. We split up when I was pregnant. I felt that if I postponed the baby until after the right woman came along and after we had established ourselves together, I might well be into the menopause.*

*In fact, it turned out that I was right not to expect a partner to appear on the scene for quite some time. It wasn't until Claire was 5½ that I met Theresa, fell in love with her and set up home with her. We've now been a family for nearly two years and I no longer think of myself as a single mother. But for five and a half years, I was on my own with Claire, and at first it was hell.*

*During that time, the one saving grace was Marie. [Marie's account follows Toni's piece.] Marie has looked after Claire at least once a week and on occasional weekends since Claire was six months old. She is an exceptional friend and has only let me down once that I can remember. If something came up and she couldn't have Claire when she'd promised, she would find another babysitter herself. This has given me valuable child-free time, so desperately needed by any single mother. But that's only a small part of Marie's involvement. What she has given Claire is just as valuable – another long-term relationship with someone who loves her. It has prevented me and Claire from developing an overly intense mother–daughter relationship. It has also been wonderful to have someone who loves Claire, with whom I can share my joy in Claire as well as my troubles. I am incredibly lucky to have had Marie in our lives.*

*Bringing up a child on my own has brought to the surface intensely painful feelings of loneliness and abandonment, whose root causes are deeper than just the outward experience of single parenting. Although it was excruciatingly painful at times, the feelings were so powerful that I could no longer escape them and I had to find strength within myself to face them. I found guidance in this through psychotherapy and Buddhism. By the time I met Theresa, I had already worked through much of my craziness, discovered some inner resources and was able to be open to her and to my friends. Ironically I had just reached a place where I was happy to be a single parent when I met Theresa.*

*These excerpts from my diary during those years give an idea of what it felt like for me to be a single mother. They are the truth, but only a partial truth. During this time, my parenting was good enough, I worked part-time and did well in my work, and I kept up many close friendships. I had fun times, but underneath . . .*

*November 1985: I can manage well but overall I feel desperately lonely. The weekends and evenings cause me to panic if I haven't arranged activities. I run away from my panic. I spend the time on the phone or watching TV. I'm constantly anxious – a tight knot in my chest. I can't pin it on anything. It seems to be the dread of being on my own. I have no control over any aspect of my life. I can't make friends, I can't clear up Claire's diarrhoea, I can't drill into the wall to put up the fireguard.*

*February 1986: I feel no connection with anyone. I don't matter in anyone's life. If I don't call people up, no one will call me. If I didn't make arrangements and invite people over, no one except Marie would come to see me. All my friends have me down on their list as a friend to see not more than once a month. I make an effort to visit with someone every day but the visits feel hollow. There must be something wrong with me. Throughout this last week, I've also had moments of intense happiness – little shivers of joy – mostly when I'm with Claire or thinking of her. She's an unbelievable treasure to me. I wouldn't be any happier living with someone. I need someone who cares about me, who's special to me.*

*April 1986: Is my sense that I make all the initiative correct or is it a screening out of the facts to fit my distorted world view? No one needs me even for practical things like shared childcare. Terrible anxiety – impotent rage – when Claire shouts her frustration, it feels like a saw cutting away at my nerves.*

*May 1987: Today I woke feeling exhausted and so weak I could hardly lift my head. It was a nightmare trying to get Claire ready. She wouldn't cooperate with me and I had no strength to be patient. People only want to spend such short stretches of time with me and then I still have so many hours to get through with no respite. I picture myself and Claire as this pathological family unit amidst these normal, happy families.*

*April 1988: I feel a great divide between the way I perceive my life and how I perceive my friends in couples with children. I fantasize about how easy it would be if a partner were involved to go out in the evening, to get help with childcare when I'm ill, to take turns staying home from work when the child is ill, etc. I do get jealous of those friends of mine who share parenting, and this sometimes influences my friendships with them. I can't stand to see both halves of a couple, whether lesbian or heterosexual, caring for their child when there's only me to do the same amount of work. I became irritable with their lack of individual competence and their constant fussing. They appear possessive and clingy to their children. Reciprocal childcare arrangements never get off the ground. Something that I need so much and that would benefit my daughter a lot is just not needed by mothers in couples. This makes me feel bitter and isolated.*

*December 1988: I feel I have no safety net and no flexibility with arrangements. More and more I rely on strangers I pay for help. Arrangements with friends are fraught with disappointed expectations. Everything is up to me – caring for my daughter, caring for my house, responsibility for my work, caring for my physical and mental health. I'm doing the best I can, but I wish I felt it was good enough. My life feels like a jigsaw puzzle. The pieces fit together very tightly. If one piece gets bigger, another has to get smaller. I just don't have the emotional energy to spend an evening on the phone being rejected while I search for a babysitter.*

*September 1989: I find it hard sometimes to even be around couples, because it's too painful for me to be reminded of how alone I am. The pain of being without a lover is an undercurrent with me. At times, I'm hardly aware of it. At other times it overflows and I can't escape it.*

*January 1992: Looking back at the last seven years, I can see how much stronger and happier I am in myself. If I had been who I am now when I got pregnant, my story would have been very different. What I have learned is that without a certain level of self-love, you can't even recognize support and love when it is offered, and nothing can fill the bottomless pit of desperation.*

● *Marie (1992)*

*I had been friends with Toni for quite a few years when she told me of her decision to have a child. I was very enthusiastic about the idea. Although I knew it would be difficult for Toni to have a child on her own, I thought the decision was very exciting. At that point in my life, I was quite wary of making a commitment to be involved with a child. As a friend I wanted to be supportive to Toni in her decision, but also had to be honest about what I felt able to offer.*

*I went along to antenatal classes with Toni and found myself becoming very excited at the prospect of a baby. Being present at Claire's birth was one of the most wonderful experiences of my life. Even though Toni's labour was long and painful, I felt very much present and involved in the birth. The moment of Claire's birth remains very vivid and alive in my memory. For me it was an intensely moving experience. Being there has made me feel very connected to her. Every year around her birthday, we look at the birth photos together and I tell her yet again the story of her being born! For me, this ritual reinforces the bond I feel we have developed.*

*When Claire was about six months old, I discussed with Toni the possibility of me having a more regular commitment to have Claire stay overnight with me once a week. By this time I felt quite sure that I wanted more involvement with her. Our relationship began to grow from this time and I could feel that Claire saw me as someone significant in her life. At first my commitment was to Toni as a friend, but gradually my feelings towards Claire developed into an independent relationship. This is because I had her for long periods (weekends as well as overnight) on my own and I got the opportunity to relate to her in my own way. All this happened because Toni was a single parent and needed support, but also because she respected and valued my relationship with Claire. She was never possessive of her daughter. In fact she positively wanted Claire to have a close bond with another adult. I think that once I made the commitment and saw that it was encouraged by Toni, I knew that it would last for ever. As long as we are living in the same country, I will always be involved with them.*

*It is a special and unique relationship. I have had the chance to feel what it is like to be a mother without the full weight of sole responsibility. There were times when she would call me 'mummy'. I would never contradict her because deep down it made me feel very happy to be called this. I feel very much part of Claire's life. In the last few years, she started describing me as her 'part-time mum'. I like that because that is what I feel towards her.*

*There were times when I was on my own with her for a whole weekend and I would feel desperately lonely and alone. It made me realize how lonely it can be being a mother. It was my sole responsibility. Only having a little child to communicate with made me realize how much I need adult company. The loneliness was so scary that it made me think that if I ever have a child, I won't do it on my own. Also seeing Toni in such a state when Claire was 2 convinced me that I would not consciously choose to go through this on my own. Sometimes it made me desperate to see how freaked out Toni was, because I didn't feel strong enough to help. She needed another adult living there. It didn't feel as if my help could ever be enough.*

*My times with Claire over the last seven years have opened up my eyes to the responsibilities involved in raising a child. Being involved with Claire has made me question my own desires to have a child. I realize there are parts of me that want to be a mother and other parts of me that feel too afraid to. Whatever I eventually decide, it will be with my eyes wide open, because I have learned a lot. And if I decide to never have a child, I hope I don't ever feel regret. Hopefully I won't, because Claire has satisfied many of my needs and given me many happy and rewarding feelings you can get from loving a child.*

### ● Bronwen (1992)

*I always thought I would have children. When I was 29, I decided to get pregnant. I was having a passionate and romantic relationship with a man but I knew that we were not going to be parents together, as he was with someone else. I tried to get pregnant with him but was unsuccessful. I only got herpes. That relationship finished quite painfully. A very close male friend had suggested we might have a baby and I really got excited by that idea, but he changed his mind. I felt I was running to a timetable, that I was on a roller coaster of just feeling that I had to do it. I was slightly worried about my age, which in retrospect seems crazy. Now I'm 37 and I'm thinking I'd better think about it in the next four years if I'm going to have another baby. But at the time I felt I just had to go ahead.*

*In a way, although I was doing it on my own, the context in which I was getting pregnant was one in which I was going to be living near a friend who also had a baby, so it didn't feel quite as alone as in fact it was. I knew that I would share a house with friends who were also going to have children, either in separate flats or together. My other best friend was trying to get pregnant and she subsequently had her own baby six months after my son, Rhys, was born. We shared a house until she moved out when Rhys was 3. This was partly because we were terribly overcrowded living in a small house. We had taken in a young woman to live with us, who then had a baby herself. I had never chosen to live alone and I'd never really taken in the implications of it just being me and him.*

*Since then, Rhys and I have had four years on our own. Now I'm so used to it, the independence and running my own show and my own family, that I don't know how I'd ever make space for someone else to come in and live with us. I feel like we're really set in our ways now.*

*My feeling is that knocking against just one adult's personality and abilities, whilst adequate, isn't the best way for a child to grow up. I think it's probably healthier for a child to be very close with more than one adult. In the absence of another adult in our family, I've made a situation arise where he has other big relationships with adults in his life. He's shown a need for that. I don't care whether it's a father figure or not. Rhys calls them his friends. These adults happen to be men because our men friends tend not to have children already. Our women friends tend to be mothers of his friends. Although he has strong relationships with them, it's not the same intensity as with an adult who's come to play with him.*

*David was his first childminder and his best friend and in some ways is like a father figure to him. When Rhys was 2, David left the country to work for nine months. That was a big change in Rhys's life and has set up quite a combative dynamic between them since. From being totally in love with David, it's now much more complicated and much more like an actual relationship with a dad. Rhys has transferred his idealizing, in-love feelings towards another man, Donald, who is a friend and plays with Rhys regularly. He really, really loves Donald, who is a wonderful bloke, and has an absolutely lovely time with him when they are together. In terms of Rhys's hierarchy of who he loves, he says he loves himself and his cousin the most, then me, then Donald. David is placed after Donald, which is partly to do with the combativeness that's developed since David left him. Rhys is actually terribly close to David – close love and hate like you get in a family.*

*Being on my own has been the toughest thing. At times the pressure of my desire to do well at work and the pressure of living in London and working full-time and trying to be a good parent has clouded my ability to really feel delight and joy in my son. Sometimes I don't really relax and play and enjoy the moment I'm in. I'm just rushing on to the next thing – minding him, tidying up, getting our things ready, doing my work. I think it has interfered with my joy in him.*

*I chose to be a single parent, so I'm not walking around with feelings of being abandoned by a partner. However, I do have some feelings of isolation and abandonment. I have had moments of pushing Rhys in a buggy across a windswept park when I have felt so abandoned. Not that I have been abandoned, but I let myself get into a situation where I was very isolated.*

*When you live on your own, there's a particular kind of pressure. You can't just let your child be. He may be playing at home quite happily, but you've got to pop out somewhere. He has to do everything with you. It isn't ideal for children or mothers. I had to go and pick up my car from the garage the other day, and it was late at night and very cold. Rhys had to wait up, get his clothes on, walk out in the dark with me for a tiny task that takes only twenty minutes. When other people are around living with you, whether they are joint parents or friends, the pressure eases up. If you run out of milk, you can go to the corner shop without having to get someone out of their pyjamas and put them in the buggy. One of you can wash up and clear up the supper while the other puts the child to bed, and then the childcare part of the day is finished, whereas when you're on your own, it's flat out – bathing, changing, dressing, bed, story, and then you still have the housework. It makes your parenting much more of a full-time job on top of your full-time employment.*

*I wouldn't let it put anybody off. I still think single parents lead the way in being a model to double parents in so many things. Firstly, single parents know that you have to have adult allies, and that you have to build up very good relationships with other adults. One adult isn't enough, but two adults aren't enough either, especially when those two adults are trying to have a relationship with each other. Time and time again, I see double parents who neglect their own relationship and don't recruit other adults into their children's lives. They do this to the detriment of their own* relationship and eventually to the detriment of their parenting, because if they're not getting on, that's tough on the children. Whereas a single parent can be quite good at having lovers and putting attention into her relationships with her lovers. I know that we need to go out and spend time alone as adults. I've had three relationships in the seven years since Rhys was born. I have probably gone out with them once a week or once a fortnight, much more than double parents do with each other. I know the relationship with the lover needs energy and time alone together.

You can tell those children whose parents are single by choice. Our children are very confident in the world. I know that my child needs more than just me, but also more than two adults. He has learned to be confident with a range of adults. I think we lead the way in building up allies and babysitters and in giving our children space to develop strong relationships with other adults.

I feel jealous but also critical of double parents – jealous of the support they have without knowing it, but critical of their preciousness and protectiveness of their children. They make such a song and dance over their children, especially two parents with their first child. They never leave the poor child alone, with the child's every need being met. I nearly killed myself trying to meet Rhys's every need, but when you see two people running around to get the right hanky to wipe the child's nose, I just feel the child needs a break from the intensity of that attention. A single parent's child doesn't have the 'luxury' of that intensity.

Although I'm a single parent, that doesn't mean that Rhys doesn't feel he has a family. He regards his family as me, my sister and brother, my sister's child and my mum. He's completely confident about that. But he also has several other families. I sometimes say to him that David and me and him are a family. We always spend weekends with my best friend and her two children and we sometimes call that our family.

I made the decision to have a child on my own because I had given up on trying to get a close relationship with another adult. But I've found that having a child doesn't stop you growing and meeting people you like and having relationships with lovers. My experience of having a child has only deepened the potential of my relationships with other adults, and has deepened my connection with my mother and my family.

# Doing it together

When a lesbian couple co-parent, they are setting out on a process which has as much potential to be challenging and exciting as it has to be fraught with difficulties. On the positive side, there are no set roles to model yourselves on, no restrictions on how to parent. You have the space to create the roles that suit your individual and joint styles. You have the potential for equality in parenting, unlike heterosexual couples who have generations of gender conditioning to contend with first. Children raised by two parents with equal power have a unique opportunity to learn about equality in relationships. The flip side of this open-endedness is anxiety and lack of clarity about just what the roles should be, and difficulty getting beyond the significance of the biological relationship. Whether the couple make the decision together to have children, or whether one or both have children from before the relationship, there is at least one partner who has a non-biological relationship to a child. How each couple defines the non-biological relationship will vary from family to family, but whatever it is, it will be new and experimental and hard for other people to understand.

This section is not meant to set out new role models for lesbian couples, but to show that everyone is struggling in their own ways to work out patterns of family relationships. The most successful co-parenting relationships are those where the partners communicate with each other about what they want and accept that parenting is a constantly changing activity, requiring continual adjustments and honesty with each other. We can't be successful all the time and it's probably best to assume that there will be rough patches.

While most co-parenting relationships are between lovers or ex-lovers, there are lesbians involved as co-parents who have never been lovers with each other. They may be friends, sisters, or women who have lived together at one time. Although their experiences are not reflected in this section, that doesn't mean that their co-parenting is any less valid or any less family than when the co-parents have been lovers.

## Just another nuclear family?

One issue that causes much confusion and pain is that of our apparent similarity to the typical heterosexual nuclear family. On the surface, a lesbian couple bringing up children together appears to be just like a nuclear family. There are two adults, with one or several children, living together and getting on with domestic life. Heterosexual friends may feel more comfortable relating to the lesbian family as if it is no different from their own. The danger in this situation lies in its complete denial of the lesbian relationship and of the uniqueness of the bond between the non-biological mother and her child. Without clarity about what kind of family it really is, the women involved can feel that they are living a lie and are invisible. In the heterosexual nuclear family, the father and mother teach by their example how men and women are meant to behave and how men and women relate to each other. Whatever role she may take on, the non-biological mother can never take on the role of father. She has neither the biological connection nor the necessary gender to teach her child what men are all about. The couple are not providing their children with role models of heterosexual behaviour. In very fundamental ways, the lesbian family is different from the nuclear family.

We can affirm and celebrate our differences from the heterosexual norm by redefining the concept of family. The legalistic definition of the family as a group of people related by blood, marriage or adoption does not apply to lesbians, or to many heterosexual people for that matter. A more real definition that includes lesbians with children as well as couples without children is that of a group of people who love and care for each other and are in committed, intimate relationships to one another. This is the concept of the family that we need to carry with us, rather than comparing ourselves with, or letting others see us as a variant of, the nuclear family.

## The non-biological mother

There are no established roles for the non-biological mother. She can take on a parental role, or the couple may decide that she has a caring role without parental responsibility. If she is a co-parent, the couple decide whether they want fifty-fifty sharing of all responsibilities or some other arrangement. While the lack of role expectations gives the woman space to create her own role, it is undoubtedly an insecure position. Her position may seem ambiguous and is bound to be discounted by others, and perhaps even by herself. She will inevitably hear her role dismissed by someone saying, 'But you're not the real mother.' Children may pick up on this lack of recognition and use it against the non-biological mother. It takes time and patience to explain the non-biological mother's role to other people and to gain acceptance for it. It is not uncommon to feel anxious, jealous and possessive and to need a great deal of reassurance. There is very little reinforcement for the validity of this role.

On the other hand, the non-biological mother's role can be very rewarding. Regardless of how other people see or define it, her position is solid and real both to herself and to the child. There may even be advantages to not having the biological connection. The co-parent may find it easier to set limits and have clearer boundaries in her relationship with the child than the biological mother can.

The legal role of the non-biological mother is discussed in Chapter 6, 'The Law'.

### What name to use?

There is no generally agreed-on name to call the non-biological mother. It seems important to have one as a way to give the role recognition. In this section, I am using the term 'non-biological mother' to make it clear who I am talking about, but it is a mouthful and does define her in terms of what she doesn't have, rather than in a more positive way. 'Co-parent' is gender neutral, which may or may not appeal to everyone. 'Co-mother' or 'foster mother' are other possibilities which are sometimes used. Some women say they are both mothers, emphasizing the social definition of 'mother'. Other women feel uncomfortable with this, as it gives no acknowledgement to the biological connection and implies there is no difference between the two mothers. It isn't easy to come up with an adequate term, but on many occasions it will be useful to have one.

### Relationships with children

When any two people parent together, they inevitably have different and unique relationships with the children. This is due partly to their separate personalities and partly to the fact that each one has different expectations of parenting, but it is also due to the importance they place on the biological connection. There is no denying the biological bond that a birth mother has with her child, but equally there is no denying the bond that grows out of the caring, intimacy and commitment to the child by the non-biological mother. Bonding comes about through intimate, caring time alone with the child, and is hindered by the lack of such time. It isn't necessarily easy to create the conditions for strengthening these bonds, nor do all women see the need for it. Some biological mothers consciously or unconsciously want an exclusive, intense relationship with their child, and may feel jealous if they see a similar bond developing with the non-biological mother. Some non-biological mothers do not want to be as involved as the biological mother, or feel unconfident of their position. Many women value the child's bonds with other adults and go to great lengths to encourage it to happen. This is just as important for many single mothers (see the section 'Doing it On Your Own'). If the couple wants the child to form a strong relationship with the non-biological mother, then time has to be made for them to develop their own unique bond. Strong bonds can be formed with older children when the partner has not been around since conception just as easily as it can with babies. The main thing is time and trust and clear communication about what each partner really wants.

## Relationships with each other

Although there is potential for equality within a lesbian couple, the power balance between the two women can be affected by many issues, such as race, class, finances, roles and personalities. When there are children born into the family, the biological connection can influence the power balance. The biological mother may feel that her commitment to parenting is deeper than that of the non-biological mother's, while the non-biological mother may feel excluded from the mother–child relationship. Or the decision to get pregnant may not be mutual and the non-biological mother may feel in a less powerful position as a result. The lack of a legal position for the non-biological mother is bound to affect the feelings of power within the relationship (see Chapter 6, 'The Law').

Just as the bonds with children are promoted by special time together, so the couple needs regular time together without children. No relationship can grow without time for intimacy. This need is often overlooked or overwhelmed by the difficulties in finding babysitters, but it is as valuable as time spent with the whole family, or the time each mother spends on her own with children (not to mention time alone).

### Getting support

Every 'normal' family has its ups and downs, including lesbian-led families. When problems come up, it is particularly hard for lesbians to know where to turn for help. Many lesbians are unable to talk about tensions and conflict within their families for fear of being thought a failure. Our mistrust of a society which attacks our right to exist and denies the validity of our families is understandable. But it is harmful if we cannot share our problems with anyone, even with other lesbians. The danger of isolation is that it creates distorted perceptions of the situation. What may be typical and even appropriate family behaviour can be interpreted by the mothers as abnormal and a sign that the family unit is sick or disturbed. The only antidote to isolation is more open communication, being willing to take risks to talk about what is going on with friends or in lesbian support groups. Parenting is not an easy activity. It has a habit of hitting you in your weakest spot. Creating support networks is as important for families led by lesbian couples as it is for women raising children on their own.

### Splitting up

It is all too common for co-parents to split up. From the biological mother's point of view, what started out as a joint activity turns into single parenthood. From the non-biological mother's perspective, she faces the very real risk of losing her child. It is at this point that she learns whether her bond with the child will be respected. While some couples split up and stay friends, for many others the split ends painfully. The bitterness and resentment women feel may make it especially hard to work out new co-parenting arrangements. Many couples do negotiate successful arrangements for shared parenting in their separate households. Others do not. Often, it is the biological mother who has more power and has the child living with her.

It is probably not wise to go to court in this situation (see Chapter 6, 'The Law'). Ideally we need a lesbian mediation service, or at least one that is not homophobic, which could help the co-parents come to some solution that works for them.

● *Rose (1992)*

*Iona and I have been together for just over five years. Even before we got together, I knew that Iona had dreams of having a child. At first, the newness of the relationship meant that I didn't take it on as my issue. It was something that Iona wanted and I celebrated that with her and encouraged her. It was too early to think that it had anything to do with me because that would have been presuming that this was a long-term relationship. A year after we got together, we made a big step in our commitment to each other when I moved down from Glasgow. It was then that I started thinking that having a baby was about both of us. During that time, there were long periods where we didn't even mention it, but it was still around. It became much more our issue when Iona started looking for a donor. That was about two and a half years after getting together. We began talking seriously then about our relationship and mine to the child when we got the first donor.*

*I do want so much to do it. I am very committed. I'm prepared to change my working patterns and to support Iona financially. I will give what I can to a child. I feel that I have a lot to contribute to creating the conditions in which a child grows up. I'm seriously planning to give a lot and make this huge life change, but I don't want to give it for no rewards. However, I'm sure there will be rewards and I welcome that.*

*Part of me is committed to doing it, but there's a bit of me that feels confused. I have been dealing with my anger about it recently. The core decision is Iona's. Iona is asking me to commit myself to something that demands so much. It's such a huge thing to ask anyone to do, especially to ask another woman. I can't think of anything in my whole life that I would ever make such a commitment to that is not fundamentally coming from me. I find that so hard. But I'm still prepared to do it, partly because I want to be with Iona. Iona is making a decision that can potentially change our whole relationship or end it altogether. The bottom line is that at the end of the day, she is saying, 'I want this child and even if I don't have you, I'm going to have the child anyway.' That's the reality of it and it is painful. It challenges me to the core. I've done* so much thinking about it that I may as well have my own child. Part of me thinks I will eventually.

We've been lovers for five years and obviously we have issues of power and control like any couple, but we've managed to work through a lot of that. We've achieved a balance in the sense that at times one of us is more powerful than the other, but that's transferable. It's fine. With Iona's decision to have a baby, we're back to a situation where Iona is very powerful and I'm very powerless. If Iona was to decide not to have a child, I would be quite happy with that. If she decides, as she has decided, that she wants to have a child, then I'll be happy with that as well. Somehow that makes me feel like a puppet. Iona's making that decision and I just have to react. But Iona might not go ahead and then I won't have that path to follow. At this early stage, where Iona is trying to get pregnant, it's hard to get over that. When Iona has the baby, then we'll have the chance to be a bit more equal, but maybe we can never be exactly equal.

To be a lesbian and a mother makes Iona more acceptable in society, but it makes me as a lesbian who isn't the mother even less acceptable than just being a lesbian. I'm creating this role for which there are no role models. Who am I? I say I am going to 'help Iona bring up the child' or I say, 'We're going to have a family.' It makes me nervous to say that. It makes me think of a man and a woman together having a family. That is so different from what we're doing. Somewhere in it all is that I'm going to be a parent. I suppose I could accept it easier if I was contributing the seed. Then it would very definitely be something that we were doing together. I don't have any part in the basic start of it all. I feel really envious of that. One solution we've come to is that I'm the one who does the inseminations. So actually I do have a role and I've given myself the title of Chief Skoosher. I was even going to get myself a T-shirt saying 'Chief Skoosher'.

It's quite new for me to be thinking about being a parent with another woman who is having a child. It's not something I learned about from my mother or that I've been reading about for years. So I'm treading quite carefully. A lot of it feels right, but when I think about society and where we are placing ourselves by doing this, it seems quite scary as well as quite exciting and positive. It almost feels too arrogant to assume the activeness of being a parent. Who am I kidding? Because what does 'parent' mean? Identity. Before, I just took it for granted that it means two people, *the mum and the dad. On the other hand, is bringing a child into the world all that makes you a mother, no matter what happens to that relationship or to that child or to you?*

*I wonder about why women have children. It's essential for me that I'm focusing on my own fundamental creativity, which I'm doing in theatre and in my drama therapy course. Iona's core creativity is in having a child. I don't know if I feel OK about it. It makes me uncomfortable because having a child seems so demanding and all-consuming in some ways. It feels like a real sacrifice, like women are giving up something of themselves to be a mother. That's how I see it as an onlooker, but I guess it's balanced because the mother is doing something creative. At least that's how I'm reconciling myself to Iona's decision. Somewhere in it, it's not just a selfless act, although she is giving up a lot. I would find it hard to think of my lover doing something so self-sacrificing. At first I thought that she should think more of herself, which was just terrible, but when I think that this is Iona's creativity, then that changes the whole picture.*

*I don't want to pretend that I'm the mother. I feel that Iona should be given the title of mother. She is the one who is going to carry the baby and give birth to it. She has made the decision, so she should be honoured with that title and I should take second place. In some ways I don't think that's very healthy for me, but I feel it's realistic. I think 'mother' is a very emotive term. It has to do with bonding and all the physical and emotional side of it. When I think of mother, I think of umbilical cords. I don't like the word 'co-parent' either. I can't really find a name. Maybe 'foster mother' would express how I feel it would actually be. It's mothering but not being a mother in the biological sense.*

*I think the biological relationship is really important while Iona is trying to conceive and is carrying the child, but when the child is born, I don't think that biological sense of mother will be so stressed. I think that it's important for the child to know who her biological mother is, but I don't think the child will have its mother and over there is Rose. If we're really serious about doing it together, then it's important that we're not saying that the biological role is the special relationship and I'm somebody else who is just there. Luckily Iona also feels like that.*

*Alongside all my fears and anxieties, I know that it's not daunting at all. It's just like any other thing which comes into your life. You adapt and change, you accommodate or you don't. Essen-*

*tially we both want to start a family, so we will find ways and it will be fine. We will celebrate it and of course there will be struggles as well. I suppose that's life.*

● *Jean (1986)*

*When my lover, Cathy, decided to get pregnant, we didn't sort it out in any depth. We didn't think about the pros and cons. She never talked to me that plainly about her feelings at the time, until after it had happened. It was something that Cathy decided she wanted to do. She hadn't even decided on self-insemination. I thought she might go and have an affair with a man. She just wanted to get pregnant, any way would do. I knew I would love Cathy's baby, but at that point I wasn't even sure what would happen if Cathy slept with a man. Would that man be involved with the baby? It was a real fear because I didn't really want him to have anything to do with us.*

● *(1992)*

*How Cathy got pregnant is very indicative of how our relationship functions. In fact, the same thing happened when I wanted to get pregnant. I remember saying, 'Right, you've got yours. My turn.' I very selfishly went ahead without a lot of discussion.*

*I had Elaine when Cathy's daughter, Alice, was 2½. It was absolute hell, with little moments of sublime joy that make it all worthwhile. Alice felt displaced. I breastfed Elaine for a long time, so that Cathy felt excluded from a relationship with Elaine. I know that I did really want this intense relationship with my baby, but I wasn't very honest about what I was doing. I didn't feel that I should or could have it. It was quite destructive. I don't think we thought about roles. The roles are quite clear when there's only one. Cathy was Alice's biological mother and Cathy was very generous with Alice in a way that I wasn't with Elaine. I fed Alice. I was very involved with her as a baby, but when Elaine came along and Alice was still very demanding, the family split down the middle, and stayed like that for quite a long time. We were all exhausted. To minimize the exhaustion and just out of ease really, I breastfed Elaine in bed because it meant that she went to sleep faster. There was this whole thing about Elaine being in bed with me and Alice getting into bed with Cathy. Alice didn't sleep through the night at 2½. She was never a good sleeper.*

I feel very different about my own child, Elaine, than I do about Cathy's daughter, Alice. My relationship with Alice is much clearer. Having your own child opens up a whole bundle of worms. The relationship between the mother and the daughter is immensely intense. I made it intense and I loved that intensity to start with, but of course it doesn't go away. It's not like a relationship that you can end. It also made me confront issues about my own childhood that I would have managed to forget. The issues around parenting that came up with Elaine because she was my child were quite different to those with Alice. They were to do with boundaries. I didn't have clearly defined boundaries in my relationship with my father, and I found it enormously difficult as a mother to Elaine to define boundaries between us. That led to a messy relationship where I was responding to Elaine's rages as if I were another child, which was completely inappropriate. That didn't happen with Alice. I had an emotional distance from Alice that didn't interfere with my love for her and made it clearer how to respond to her.

It was relatively easy being a family of two adults and one child, but as soon as Elaine came along, we felt like two exhausted single parents who happened to be living together. During the baby stage, when they are very demanding, it didn't seem to make a lot of difference having two adults. As they get older, it does get easier. But having two kids is twice as hard as having one. When one of us wants to go off and give the other partner space, there are two children to take. It's very easy to go off with a 7-year-old on your own. It's not the same taking a 7-year-old and a 4-year-old on your own.

Until Elaine was about 3, we had a very difficult time, but it is becoming much easier now. My relationship with Elaine is less intense. After the first few years when Alice behaved like a typical jealous sibling, hating the baby and not being able to bear her, now there is an immensely strong bond between them and they get on really well. It has made life so much easier. They both get up in the morning and play together. We can lie in bed for hours on weekends. When they were babies, that's something we never thought we would have in our lives again. We thought it would just go on and on and on. We have emerged from that time as a strong unit and as four separate individuals with very strong relationships with each other.

At the moment, the relationship between me and Cathy is very strong and the relationship we have with the girls is better than it ever has been. But we've had very bad patches. We've rowed in front of the girls and seen how destructive that is for them. All of our problems can be traced to a breakdown in communication, compounded by exhaustion. We just stop talking about the important things. Cathy tries to initiate discussions but it's fear that stops me talking. The fear is that if we talk, we will wreck it, and I want it to continue. We know that we can keep going. We've been together for fifteen years. We know that we're actually very good about being a household and that we're all very fond of each other. I'm very frightened of delving any deeper than that. If we talk and reveal things, then I fear that we'll no longer be in control, and things could explode. Whereas I'm quite good at the superficial maintenance – keeping things ticking over, like cooking, shopping, thinking ahead – I'm not very good at major overhauls. As I get older I become less frightened of experiencing the pain as well as the pleasure of intimacy, and also realize that we just have to go through it together. The base-line is that we love each other and our children, but we also have to work hard to keep it all going.

I'm very pleased that Alice and Elaine have had to grow up in a larger unit than a lot of single parents have. They've had to adjust to the dynamics of four people in a household instead of two or three. Also neither of them is the sole focus of two adults, which I think is actually very difficult for a child. It's not as big a family as Cathy would like. I think she would like more children. I wouldn't want any more because physically we're too old. We started too late. There are other things I want to do with my life now that I've got through the baby bit and have more energy.

Over the years I have realized how particularly stressful it is to be lesbians bringing up kids. We live as a family unit in a small, friendly street full of family houses. We have close heterosexual friends who are bringing up their children in nuclear families, with whom we have much in common in terms of the day-to-day parenting. But we are not what we appear to be. Our incomes are much lower. We are not homeowners and our lesbian relationship has very little in common with the relationships of our heterosexual friends. So when Clause 28 identified 'pretend families', it hit a raw nerve. We know we are different, but in order to be supportive to us, 'real' nuclear families tend to overlook the differences and they 'pretend' we are just like them.

*The other thing I find stressful about lesbian parenting is an enormous pressure not to talk about how awful things can be. There are issues that I feel that we mustn't talk about, like violence towards the children. I feel that we can't be completely open because we should be doing it better than heterosexuals. We've set this up. We've done it ourselves. We're going to do it perfectly. We're not going to fail. I think I've internalized that pressure. That puts us under as much if not more pressure than heterosexual families, which makes me wonder why we berate ourselves about our parenting!*

*Sometimes I'm envious of lesbians who have children on their own, because they appear to have more time to themselves. Single parents have to be far more organized about childcare and seem to make more effort to involve other adults with their children. It's very easy to be careless when there's two of you and to rely on each other too much, but this puts a great strain on the relationship. It's easy to go out separately but harder to go out together.*

*Recently a young lesbian said to me, 'I realize I'm in a very privileged position. I don't have children and I can offer help to lesbians who have children.' I nearly wept. I had not heard that in ten years. When I got involved in women's liberation, I was always helping out heterosexual feminists with their kids. The consciousness around being a mother and how mothers were oppressed in heterosexuality was really high on the agenda. We thought, 'Poor women, what awful lives. I'm a lesbian and I've got more time. I must babysit for free.' Now you're a lesbian mother and other lesbians say, 'It's your choice.' I didn't turn around to heterosexual feminists and say, 'You didn't have to fuck a man. You didn't have to get married.' Lesbians are not seen as being oppressed as mothers. At the moment, I feel so grateful that if another lesbian or gay adult shows any interest in my children, I could hug them. I think it's awful that I feel that desperate.*

*Even though we've had rough patches, in fact we do function as a unit very well and I adore both girls enormously. They're good fun. We have a lot of laughs, the four of us. There are in-family jokes. There are roles that we take – Elaine is the clown, which is common with youngest siblings. Most of all, those girls give an enormous amount to us. Our relationships with them are getting better and stronger as they get older and we're able to discuss issues and our views of the world. You don't expect this* when you have babies. It's wonderful. You can talk about issues like homelessness with a 7-year-old. I find it very exciting. I'm really looking forward to them getting older.

● *Shaheen (1992)*

As I was getting to the age of about 33 or 34, I could see my fertile years slipping away. I was becoming more and more aware of the fact that I wanted to be involved with bringing up a child. At that point, it didn't necessarily have to be my own child. But as time wore on, I could see that the simplest thing would be for me to have my own child because I had no way of knowing whether my girl-friend, Jackie, would get pregnant or, if we split up, whether I would ever meet someone else who had a child. The surest way of guaranteeing your involvement with a child is to have one yourself. It wasn't a decision that I made overnight. When I finally decided that I was going to have my own child, Jackie also wanted to have a child. She was younger than me so she started first. It took her a while to get pregnant and then she miscarried very early on. She was quite put off by the experience and was very down. Time was marching on for me so I decided that I would get going.

We both knew that we had each decided to have babies in our own right, for ourselves, not just because we were in a relation-ship and had each other's support. Our decisions were not depen-dent on the relationship being in existence. But obviously being in a reasonably safe, secure, long-term relationship was one of the major factors which made me think that this was a good condition to have a child in. By the time I decided to have a baby, Jackie and I had been together for about four years. However, my relationship with Jackie was not in mint condition when I started to go about the process of having a child.

Despite our difficulties, Jackie really stood by me during my pregnancy. I was very ill during the pregnancy. I was living on a knife edge because I thought that I was going to lose the pregnancy. I bled for the first few months and I had to stay flat on my back. During those months, I had to be walked around the park every night to get exercise and I had to be fed. Jackie did all that. I felt completely useless. I couldn't do anything. As soon as I got up, I was sick. After the fourth month, I was fine until at six months I bled again, so I had to stay in hospital for a week. After that, everything was OK until I went into labour. I had a terrible labour.

*After 41 hours, he was delivered by Caesarean. I don't think I could have done it without Jackie's support.*

When I was trying to get pregnant, I didn't in a million years think that when Anton was still a baby, we would split up. I would never have had a child if I was going to be alone. It wouldn't have been my choice to be a single parent. Even though I was living in the real world and knew that the relationship could break up at some point, I never thought that it would break up when Anton was so young and so demanding. It had been up and down for many months but it was still a real shock when it came. It took a long time for her to make the break and she felt very bad about doing it, but nevertheless she did it. I was left with the child and holding down a full-time job. Jackie said that if it hadn't been for Anton, we would have split up a lot sooner. By the time she left, we had lived together for six years.

I found it very hard to get used to the idea of being a single parent. At first I was paralysed. My whole world had turned completely upside down. My life had to be restructured to cope on my own. Everything doubled – the rent, bills, all the expenses. I found it quite lonely.

We went to the housing association and asked if they could rehouse us separately, but we had to stay living together until they could rehouse us, and it was hell on earth for a long time. After about three months, Jackie just had to go. She stayed with a friend. We couldn't bear it. I had to stay there on my own until they rehoused me. It was a very big flat with loads of memories that I wanted to put behind me.

Jackie is committed to Anton. She gives me an allowance every month for him and she has him alternate weekends and two nights a week. He's got a home with her. This is his home but he has a bed here and a bed there. That's been going on for the last year. There are hiccups but on the whole it does seem to work.

It has taken us a really long time and a lot of hard effort to work things out since we split up. We've found it very hard to get on. I've been all right but Jackie has been very bitter. She has found it really difficult to communicate with me. Sometimes she's very off-hand with me. She doesn't want to be my friend. It's really hard when you're trying to share a child not to be friends. I feel I have to keep making the effort for his sake. Now and then Jackie gets to a point where she can't cope, which means that she can't have Anton. That blows the whole 'sharing the care' arrangement. That has *happened a couple of times. It might be for a few weeks or a month and then it's OK. But she wants to maintain her commitment.*

Anton has a very strong relationship with Jackie which will be very beneficial in the future. I had him when I was in a relationship with her. She is the other mother to all intents and purposes. She's been involved since the word go, but she's got no rights. She does worry that I will leave London and take him, but I wouldn't do that. I think that would be very unfair to her and to Anton. Jackie would be absolutely heart-broken if she lost him, and I think that it would be a great loss to him too. I did have my doubts about her once when she didn't see that much of him for three months. I do realize that if she did disappear for any reason, Anton would get over it. But I think it's important that we work it out and that's what I'm aiming to do.

He doesn't call her mummy. He calls her Jackie. She wanted me to be mummy and her to be Jackie so that he wouldn't get confused. Even though she really is his mother, she doesn't like the label. I think that she thought that we can never have an equal place for the simple reason that I was the one who gave birth to him. He sometimes gets us confused. When he's spent a weekend with her, he comes home calling me Jackie. It's just a momentary lapse. He will call her mummy but he'll correct himself very sharply.

Jackie is very threatened by my new lover, Ellen. Ellen and I have been together for nine months. It doesn't seem to matter what I say to Jackie or how much I try to convince her that no one could take over her role. No one else could possibly mean to Anton what Jackie means to him. She was there when he was born. She's got a relationship with him that no one else will ever have. She's not convinced.

Ellen wants to have a child and I'm really pleased. She would like the child to have contact with the man. It would be very unequal for us. Her child would have a father and Anton wouldn't. But Anton would have three mummies. If Ellen does have a child and we do stay together, we would like to live together. Then it would be very weird because Anton would be off with Jackie half the week and I would probably spend more time with Ellen's child than my own. Ellen said she wouldn't see herself as co-parenting Anton because that's Jackie's role, but if we did all live together, I think his relationship with Ellen would change. My mind boggles when I think of all the things to be considered and discussed.

I've come out of a long, dark tunnel now. I was in the pits a *year ago and now things are much more in my control. Anton goes to full-time nursery. I work four days a week. I'm living in a much more manageable place with a garden. When I encounter other women just starting out on this road, I think, 'Thank God, I've done it and it's over.' I'm so pleased that I've got Anton, who is a lovely boy, and that everything is falling into place, but there's no way I'd ever go through that again. I have toyed with the idea of having another child because I never wanted Anton to be an only child. But I eliminated that thought pretty rapidly.*

*I've got friends who are trying to have a child now. I can never say often enough to them that it's going to change every single aspect of their lives. It does come as a shock. You can't go to the toilet on your own, you can't wash on your own. You can't do anything. There's always that child hanging around you wanting your attention, wanting something. You can feel like tearing your hair out and chucking him out of the window. Parenting isn't natural. I don't think it's something women are born for. You hear people say that staying home and looking after your child is natural. It's a load of rubbish. It's a skill that is learned and which should be taught at school.*

*I've learned that you shouldn't underestimate what having a baby is going to take out of you. So many women do. I was one of them. It's vital to have a good support network or at least one person who can give you support, because you're going to need an awful lot of it. It doesn't have to be a partner, but it's got to be long lasting and someone you can trust. It is so important to go through it with someone and not to be alone.*

### ● *Paula (1991)*

*When I was in my twenties I decided I wasn't going to have a child. But I got very broody, almost obsessive when I was 30. I don't think I thought about it very much. I'm not the sort of person who thinks about things much. I tend to go straight in. I only knew one lesbian who was inseminating at the time I was seriously thinking about it, but I knew lesbians who had children from marriages who were saying, 'Don't do it! You're mad.'*

*When I first met Nicole I was already pregnant and I had all the anxieties around whether she would want to know. Some of the circles we moved in didn't encourage or foster the idea that lesbians could choose to have children. It seemed to be more acceptable for lesbians to have had children from marriages. Shortly afterwards I had a miscarriage. I always made it clear to Nicole that I was going to get pregnant again, and I started trying soon after I had the miscarriage. She was very involved in the inseminations and was always there. We used a friend as a go-between. I got pregnant in the second month. I always felt that Nicole was quite excited about the prospect of being involved. It was all very vague, as if somehow things would just work out, but we hadn't really talked about her parenting role. Part of the problem was that I didn't really want to talk about the pregnancy until I was five or six months pregnant in case I lost it.*

*Because of problems where I was living, I moved in with Nicole in short-life housing when I was about eight months pregnant. I suggested it and it seemed like a good idea at the time. I was panicking because the women I had been living with had long-term plans that didn't really include me. I felt I was going to be left on my own with a young child and I was scared. Nicole and I went through this whole thing that if it didn't work out, then it didn't work out. It was quite fun living together. Even though there were tensions around housing, we felt we were doing everything together. It was a challenge. Eventually we got housed together in a permanent lesbian co-op. We moved in three days before Tara was born. When I came out of hospital, the house was all newly decorated. All we had to do was move our furniture in and personalize it. Even at that point, we still hadn't talked about things.*

*Up to that point Nicole had been in and out of temporary jobs doing unskilled work. She was trying to look for a permanent job, which she eventually found. She started work in a very demanding job in a children's home six weeks after I had the baby. There were lots of demands on her plus the demands of coming home to a miserable girlfriend and a crying baby. It was a recipe for disaster. It was very difficult because she had come from a working-class background and hadn't had many opportunities. Here was a job that claimed to open up all sorts of doors for her. At that time, that's just what she needed, but it meant she had to give up other things. It was very bad timing. That's when the resentment built up and I thought she didn't give a stuff for me and Tara. One time Tara and I were sick with flu and she wouldn't take a day off work to look after us. I had to ring up a friend to help me out. I used to say that she loved that job more than she loved us.*

*It was like we were married. We shared the same bedroom.*

*The baby was always there. We didn't have any privacy. We didn't have a sex life. She was the one going out to work and I was the one staying at home. I had lots of time on my own with Tara, so when Nicole came home I wanted her to spend time with me. I expected Nicole to come home from work and take Tara off, take her out of the house, change her, feed her, do the shopping, do the cleaning, entertain me. She had to do sleep-overs. She would come home 24 hours later really tired, and it was too much for her to see me or the baby. She wanted to be on her own. I think we wanted different things and I don't really think we talked about it.*

*We initially split up about six months ago, and then we got back together again, but she is moving out now. I think we were both scared to admit that it wasn't working. I don't know what happened. I think we just didn't talk. I had an expectation of her that was unrealistic. I will always say that Nicole did do her share at the beginning. We would always take it in turns to get up and feed Tara. No matter how much she hated it, she would do it. But once she got her job, I kept feeling like she was in a privileged position. I never looked at what it was like for her. I felt a lot of resentments.*

*She said to me when we split up that she didn't want to see me for three months and that involved not seeing Tara. At first I accepted it, and then I got really angry and I refused to accept it. Because whatever happens between me and her, it shouldn't affect Tara. I told her that if she's going to be a parent, she can't suddenly decide one week she is and the next she's not. It doesn't work like that. I've always said to her that I can't walk away from Tara. At the end of the day, that's where the difference lies. It's the degree of responsibility. There's lots of issues around that for her, like the fact that she doesn't get any recognition as a parent, that I've always taken responsibility and never given her any. I don't think that's always true. She keeps saying to me now that her job is not designed for people who have children. If she'd known that at the time, perhaps she would have considered something else. I've chosen to take a part-time job, at least until Tara's a bit older. When we were still together the second time around, Nicole said she was looking for another job that didn't involve sleep-overs. But by that point it was too late.*

*In a way I got a lot stronger from all the times I had to cope. Now I do nearly all the childcare. It's down to me. It's a sense of relief in a way. I can just get on with it.*

*Tara seems OK about not seeing Nicole as much. She misses her and always asks where she is. But there's nothing unusual about her not seeing Nicole for two or three days, because of Nicole's working. I'm hoping that Nicole will see her at least once a week, which will be a bit different for Tara, but I think she'll adjust. I don't think she'll have any problems.*

*If I get involved with anybody else, I'm very wary about them getting involved with Tara. I don't want them to usurp Nicole's position, even though I don't know what her position is at the moment. I don't necessarily want a new lover to have a parenting relationship with my child. I know a couple of women who have had relationships since their children have been born, and it's been very hard on their children. The children get involved, then the person decides to leave and doesn't see the children for months. You can't treat children like that. In fact that's the way I was treated when I was a child. My dad left and I have this real thing about it. I don't want Tara growing up with a sense of loss. I would be very careful about other relationships. Unless I really fell madly in love with someone and it was going to be a total involvement, I think I would try to keep it separate. It sounds sensible but actually I haven't been very sensible.*

*Nicole never felt comfortable about Tara calling her mummy because she felt that I was her mummy. If Tara wanted to call her mummy, then that would be OK with Nicole. I don't think Nicole is her mum. It's a funny distinction but I do see Nicole as a parent. It doesn't feel comfortable to me to call Nicole Tara's mum because mum means the primary carer, the one who gave up things to have her. I gave up working. I gave up some choices.*

*The advice I would give to lesbian couples who are thinking about having children is to remember that you're not in a heterosexual relationship and do not have to live up to a heterosexual image of the family. You don't need to think that you have to perform in a certain way. If you're not getting your needs met, then you have to say. If your needs part at any point, you have to say. Nicole used to say to me that if she were a man, she would be getting away with murder. I used to say that she's not a man. We have to remember that we're independent women and we can still change it at any point. It doesn't have to be for ever, and if it is and it works out, that's fine. If it doesn't, it doesn't. I just don't think we should live up to any sort of myths, such as if you're a couple with children, you have to stay together or else you're going to do the child's head in. People always ask how it's affecting Tara and say how terrible it is. Nicole used to say we mustn't argue in front of Tara. I felt we had to closet her. I think it's better for her to know reality, and not to be cushioned. It did affect her, but she can cope with that. She can cope with emotions. Children aren't dolls to be put away. That's another myth – that children shouldn't see that we are real people. We can have space and time away from each other and that's all right. We don't stop functioning as individuals just because you're in love with someone and caring for a small child.*

### ● Kath (1986, Ruth born in 1985)

*I couldn't handle my partner Judy getting pregnant by sleeping with a man. If I was going to co-parent this child, then that meant I was going to co-parent from conception. I had to have everything to do with it. Some of that is about reassurance. I feel very easily threatened, taking this on as a non-biological mother. A biological event in it can really threaten it. There's something there that I wouldn't be part of. All decisions were made together. We decided together when we were both ready to have children and other things about the donor, like anonymity.*

### ● (1992)

*Judy and I chose together to create a new person to introduce into the world. We have a clarity between us that Ruth is our child. Our motivations might have differed but they were equal. I do not want to be pregnant, nor has that ever been a major fascination for me. Nevertheless I am a parent. Wanting to be pregnant and wanting to be a parent are two very different things. OK, so there's one obvious connection. The former does tend to lead to the latter, but it is no more or less inevitable than heterosex being the only way to conceive.*

*One of the most difficult things has been dealing with other women's (mainly lesbians') inability to get their heads and their words around the wholeness of our family. It makes me feel angry rather than anything else. It feels like I'm being dismissed. I do as much for Ruth. I have as many sleepless nights. I have washed as many nappies. I take as much of the responsibility as Judy does. It makes me furious when people ask which one of us is her reall proper mother. The short reply is that we both are.*

Given that, I did have to recognize, sometimes painfully, from early on that Judy's biological relationship to Ruth was more significant than I had thought it might be. The months of breast-feeding were hard. I was jealous and felt I had to change and wash more nappies to compensate, had to wake up to fetch her for a feed in the night even if I couldn't deliver it. This became easier after the first few months when we moved on to mixed bottle/breastfeeding, which worked well for us despite the orthodoxy which says that bottlefeeding can distract babies from the breast.

Ruth knows whose tummy she grew in and whose breasts she sucked, but she still calls me mum. If we're both around, she will address us by name if she has a need she particularly wants one of us to address. If she isn't fussy, she will shout the generic 'mum' and deal with whichever one of us responds. Sometimes I am the interloper between her and Judy and she wants me out of the way. Those moments are sometimes painful, sometimes irritating, but they come with the turf, new and unbroken, and I/we have to live them through. The rough bits of the journey are eased by the clarity of the contract between me and Judy. Neither of us is interested in sole parenthood or in building in the biology. We note the significance of the biological relationship and then get on with the job of parenting. Ruth's relationship to both of us is equally strong but different. It's frankly impossible to sort out what, if any, has to do with a biological link between Ruth and Judy and what is due to us being different people. Sometimes it has been a source of stress, but we're just working our way through it. All of our relationships are growing and changing all the time.

It was clear from Ruth's early days on the planet that in order to both be active parents, we had to actively resist heterosexual models of carving up the week and the sheer graft involved in bringing up a young child. After a disastrous attempt (for her and us) to involve a childminder in our childcare arrangements, we realized that what we both wanted was to share childcare and work part-time. Giving up the security of full-time work was scary but also a privileged choice we were able to make, given we had jobs in the first place and flexible ones at that. What this meant in practice was that we both had individual extended time with Ruth, time together as a family and equally precious time out in the world functioning as individuals. Thus we both experienced the ups and downs of parenting a baby/toddler/child without the isolation and insanity of doing it full-time.

*This did mean, however, that until relatively recently (the last year) we have had very little space alone together. Now we get out once a week. After six years of investing so much energy in parenting, our relationship was suffering, but once we recognized what we needed to do and did it, life improved for all of us. We'd advise other women not to leave it so long. Look after yourselves as well as your children!*

*Inevitably two adults bringing up a child bring their own styles and ideas of parenting, and as you go along, it's amazing what surfaces from your own past and how these sometimes clash. We've generally found, however, that we can maintain our different styles and relationships with Ruth, but have agreed common approaches to major issues, routines and a common direction. The common ground is what has held us together in our own relationship and it's that which underpins the atmosphere of our family. We sometimes have, for example, differences around issues of discipline, which we have had to confront and negotiate, but we have a common philosophy of treating Ruth as a whole person, capable of understanding the answer to any question she chooses to ask, and that she has rights within our family.*

*She is aware of our different styles and exploits them to her advantage. She knows exactly which of us to ask for what, and when. On the other hand, she has benefited from our different strengths and the different relationships she has with each of us. I've taught her to swim, ride her bike and bake bread while Judy has taught her to ice-skate, sew and plant bulbs.*

*Our sub- but nearly nuclear family unit works well for us. On the surface it looks like a heterosexual model of the family. But there are very major differences, in terms of the real collectivity with which we organize our family, and the fact that we are lesbians. I feel resentful of heterosexuals assuming we are just like them and ignoring what might happen between us when Ruth goes to bed. It makes me feel that our lesbian family is invisible.*

# Chapter five

# The Children

## The sex of your child

THERE is a widely held but erroneous belief that donor insemination produces more boys than girls. This isn't true of donor insemination, either in a clinic or by self-insemination. There is the same ratio of boys to girls as there is from sexual intercourse. You can't generalize from small samples. A cluster of five or six boys conceived by self-insemination in the same year doesn't prove anything. When a group of us sat down and added up all the self-inseminated babies we knew of personally, we counted twenty-two boys and twenty-four girls. It may be that there is a slight difference, but so far it looks like a 50:50 ratio.

Many women have a preference for their child to be one sex rather than the other. This is very common and is certainly not limited to lesbians desiring girl babies. Heterosexual women are free to express their preferences without fear of anyone passing judgement on their suitability for parenthood. A lesbian takes the risk of facing strong reactions if she is open about her wishes. Not all lesbians do prefer girls. Those that do may be accused of immaturity or of hating males by straight society.

Lesbians who prefer boys or who have boy children may come up against the hostility of some women in the lesbian community. Unfortunately there are still many childless lesbians (and even some mothers) who make life in the lesbian community very uncomfortable for mothers of boys. As more and more lesbians take advantage of donor insemination and have children, these attitudes are bound to change. At the moment, women getting pregnant often change their circle of friends and create support networks with women who care for children, biological mothers or not. It is hard enough raising a child without having to contend with hostility over something you had no influence over.

Many women have expressed profound worries about the implications of trying to select the sex of your child. If it were possible to do on a large scale, it could lead to an imbalance in the ratio of males to females. Given the attitudes towards women in most societies in the world, this would probably mean that there would be more men than women. Even on a smaller scale, what would be the consequences to the lesbian community if it were possible to choose the sex of children reliably? Would lesbians who chose to have boys or who didn't actively choose to have girls end up ostracized?

On an individual level, the consequences of strongly desiring one sex are very serious and need to be considered before you start trying. In her book, *Considering Parenthood* (see Appendix A), Cheri Pies describes a useful exercise for exploring your feelings about the sex of the baby. Ask yourself how you feel about raising a boy or a girl. Imagine that you have just given birth and that your baby is a girl. Allow yourself to observe your reactions without judging them or suppressing any. Sit and think for a few minutes or write your thoughts down as they come. Do the same, imagining that you have just had a boy. Having a preference doesn't mean that you won't love a child of the opposite sex. But if you aren't prepared to have a child of one sex, then you might not want to be a mother yet.

There have been claims that a woman can increase her chances of conceiving a boy or a girl by various methods. A lot of scepticism greets these claims and there are no reliable studies showing that they work. One claim is that the timing of inseminations is important, but one carefully conducted US study showed that this isn't true. This study, which is described in Robert Winston's book *Getting Pregnant*, found that the sex of 1,188 children who were conceived after one insemination at a clinic could not have been predicted by the time in the woman's menstrual cycle when the insemination was done. Various other methods have been proposed such as vaginal douching, diets and sperm separation. None claims to be 100 per cent effective. Any woman trying one of them must feel strongly enough to make the extra effort at the same time as she remains open to having a baby of the other sex. Just as important is the fact that all the methods have the effect of delaying or inhibiting conception. You are likely to be trying for longer to get pregnant using these methods.

### ● *Linda (1986)*

When I had the amniocentesis, I think they would have told me the sex but I didn't want to know. I thought I would have a surprise. I started off actually wanting a girl. And then I thought, 'Oh my God! I can't just go on like this, because it may be a boy.' So Margaret (my lover) and I got really psyched up to having a boy. We got this name for a boy, and we got the boy all sussed out. Just before she was born, in that last week, a nurse thought it was a girl and she said something. I felt completely unprepared for a girl when she was born.

### ● Shaheen (1992)

When I told all my friends that I wanted to get pregnant, a typical reaction was, 'What are you going to do if it's a boy?' A lot of people think you'll panic if you have a boy. There's this myth that lesbians hate men. I suppose I did go through a stage of hating men when I first came out as a lesbian, when I was very young, but I came out of that years ago. I didn't mind whether it was a boy or a girl. I fully expected to have a boy. It was no shock to me when he was born. As a mother of a boy, it's my responsibility to bring him up to know that women are not objects to be used and abused. I look on it as being something very positive. It's nice to think I'm bringing up a boy who will be a man that has had a non-sexist upbringing. He is being brought up in a different lifestyle. I think it's very important to say that to people. Lesbians shouldn't just have babies because they want to have girls. I think it's terrible to use sex-selection methods.

### ● Cathy and Jean (1986)

#### Cathy

I don't believe in doing anything to try to influence the sex of the child. I think it's morally wrong. I think that you're going to have what you're going to have and that you shouldn't try and interfere. I think you have to take the risk, that's all part of getting pregnant.

I didn't allow myself to hope I'd have a girl. I never said I wanted a girl or I wanted a boy. I always said I was pretty sure I *was going to have a boy. I was in some way working on accepting having a boy during the pregnancy. I became convinced it was a boy and I was happy about that. It was a nice surprise when it was a girl. Now I feel very lucky to have a girl, especially as she gets older. And I feel very hopeful about the future relationship with a girl. I know I would love a boy. But their maleness makes things more difficult.*

### Jean

*At the moment I'd argue against that, because I feel that I've got to keep my mind completely clear of that sort of bias and prejudice because I want to get pregnant.*

### Cathy

*It's not a bias and a prejudice. I think it's just being realistic really. Perhaps it's better to really talk about it before you have the boy instead of it being rather a shock.*

### Jean

*In New Zealand, I saw lesbian mothers with boys, 11-year-old and adolescent boys, and they had very lovely, close relationships.*

### ● Mary (1986)

*If I'd had the choice I would have chosen a girl child, but I decided to get pregnant knowing full well I was just as likely to have a boy. I did use a sex-selection method for about one month, but then I gave it up because I thought it wasn't for sure anyway. I still regret not having a daughter. I've got an incredible amount of strength through being involved in feminist things – there's a set of ideas and principles which have been incredibly important to me and which I can identify with as a woman. I would like to have been able to share that with my children. I feel disappointed that I don't have the possibility of having that closeness around a shared oppression.*

*What I have to do with the boys is make it very clear where my support for them as children lies and, without putting them down as individuals, make it clear that they are part of a sex that has power in this world. I want them to be aware of that so that they won't use that power over women. I constantly talk with them about sexism. I feel I often have to play a negative role with boys – teaching them how not to do things. I spend a lot of time talking with the boys about issues of power and privilege in society. For example, how as white people we are relatively privileged compared with many others. I think that having a lesbian as a mother also helped them to understand how those other oppressions work.*

*There's a lot more fun to be had in encouraging girls. There are other children in my life and a couple of girls who I am close to. One thing that has changed since I've had children is that I have so many friends with children. I have confidence that I always will have children around me, including girls. In some ways, I'd love to go through giving birth again, having another child and learning about a whole new little person, but it's been a lot of hard work and I don't think I want to start again really.*

### ● Pat (1986)

*I read the books on how to do it to get a girl. And you do it two days before or something. By the second month, I thought, 'Oh no, I want a baby.' I didn't care. I wasn't really that bothered. I would have like to have had a girl, but only because I had Dean and he's a boy, not because I wanted a girl politically or because I was a woman. But I was really glad I had the girl in the end. It was great. I was unprepared for a girl. I was so shocked. Especially as they say, if you have a baby through AID (DI), it's always a boy. That's the myth, isn't it. People I'd known about had boys by AID as well.*

*But I wouldn't have been disappointed if it had been a boy, because of the way I felt about it by the end. My sister was disappointed and she's heterosexual. She's got two boys and she really wanted a girl. When the second boy was born, she was very upset and cried a lot. Now you would think he was her favourite in a way, but at the time she was very disappointed.*

### ● Sheila (1992)

*When I was pregnant, I did want a girl, although I was happy to have a boy as well. Very quickly after he was born, it didn't matter at all. There was a lot of anti-boy feeling in the early*

1980s *when he was little. I remember letters in the* London Women's Liberation Newsletter *about how they didn't want to have boys at crèches. There were things we couldn't go to with boys, even little tiny babies. It's not the same nowadays. We don't even have crèches any more. Recently I haven't had any hassle from lesbians about having had a boy, because I have not put myself in any situations where I would. It's nice having a boy, because it makes you challenge all that stuff. I was once a bit of a separatist but no longer. Now I really think the personality of the child and whether you get on is much more important than their sex.*

### ● Judy (1986)

*I was in a 'SI for Girls' group [a group which met to learn about ways to conceive girl babies] before the other SI group I was in was set up. I wasn't into the idea of trying for girls because I felt that, in order to decide to get pregnant, you have to deal with the uncertainty of the sex of the child. Having carried a child for four months, then to have amniocentesis and have a very late abortion seemed impossible for me and difficult for any woman. As far as I know, none of the women in the 'SI for Girls' group did get pregnant. The group was very useful in starting to sort out the donor screening stuff and it investigated all the ways in which women could affect the sex of the fetus – such as douching, timing of conception, diet, centrifuge sperm – and found out none was reliable. All were controversial.*

*When I was pregnant, women often asked me if I wanted a boy or girl, and how I would deal with having a boy. I said I didn't mind. This was confirmed when I gave birth. The baby was lying on me for ten minutes before the midwife said, 'She's a girl.' It really didn't matter.*

## Communicating with children

Women who choose self-insemination as a conscious and positive act want their children to know that self-insemination is a normal way to get pregnant, that the kinds of family they are growing up in are as nurturing and loving as any, that their lives are complete without a father figure and that they were very much wanted and planned. The children also have to be prepared for the hostility and disapproval they may face from prejudiced and ignorant people.

Of course, what you tell them depends on what there is to tell. There are no right or wrong choices, but there are consequences of each choice. If you used an anonymous donor, there will be certain answers you cannot give to your child. If the donor is known to you, it may actually be harder to explain his role, or his role may change over time. What you have to tell is likely not to be static. During your child's life, lovers may come and go, the donor's role may go through different phases, your sexual identity may change, you may start off single and later start a relationship or vice versa.

Throughout all this, your child is growing up and trying to make sense of the world. The act of telling children is not over in one session. It is part of a continuous process of two-way communication. The younger they are when you start telling them, the less likely they are to pick up society's homophobia. Children conceived by self-insemination to lesbian mothers have lived with no other reality and in theory should grow up accepting their family as the norm. But there are many other influences on children, even very young ones. They will inevitably be exposed very early on to propaganda about heterosexuality and what is considered a 'normal' family. You have to tell them what is appropriate for their age and level of understanding. It is best to make your explanations simple, straightforward and matter-of-fact. There will be times when they can hear you and times when it is best to leave it. Telling them what it means to be lesbian, about self-insemination, and about donors is a long-term process. Like any other information you give them, you have to tell them again and again. It won't sink in after one telling.

Children will learn not just what we tell them but what we convey to them indirectly and unconsciously. It is not just a matter of choosing the right words and the right timing. Children's reactions are influenced not only by their age but by the approach you take. If you feel positive about your sexuality and your choice to have a fatherless family, your child is much more likely to feel all right about it. You will be giving them a model of positive self-esteem. If you don't feel positive about what you have done and who you are, you will have a much harder time putting across a positive, affirming message to your child. It will also be much more painful for you to handle any negative reactions from your child. You may find that you thought you were clear about your choices until you are faced with your child's grief and rage; at which point, you may suffer from guilt and uncertainty. There is precious little validation for choosing to be a lesbian mother or a single mother from society. Each woman has to do her own validating for herself, but equally important is the confirmation that we can give each other. We have consciously to create our own support networks that affirm our choices to have children in this way. If you have this in your life or at least know that you are not the only one, your communication with your child will be that much clearer, more confident and less ambiguous.

Nevertheless, no matter how positive you are, you cannot control your child's reactions. Not only is your child a separate person with their own feelings and thoughts, but their position in the family is completely different from yours. They haven't chosen this family structure in the way you have. They may feel a sense of loss or anger at you or towards the donor. They may feel hurt that the donor is not interested in them. They may complain that they didn't choose to be different. Hopefully they will eventually learn that nobody chooses their families and that a good many families are different in one way or another.

Every mother will have her own ways of helping her child understand her reasons and of giving the child space and permission to react. It can be very painful for a mother to see that she has caused her child's suffering. We so much want our children to be happy that we are often prepared to do nearly anything to take away their disappointment, frustration or grief. If you can listen to your child express whatever they feel without being thrown by it and without denying it, then you are giving your child something very valuable – the message that painful emotions can be endured, that they do not destroy you.

It is fairly inevitable that children will ask about their fathers. It's impossible to know whether the desire for knowledge about the biological father is a result of social pressures or whether it would occur in a society where little significance was placed on the role of fathers. Many people who have been adopted feel strongly that they have a right to know their biological parents. Some adults in the USA who were conceived by donor insemination have formed a group demanding their right to know the donors. Wherever the desire comes from, SI children will want to know. They usually become intensely interested around the ages of 3 to 5, especially after they have been told the biological facts of life and have met a few children with fathers. They ask questions like, 'Who is my daddy? Why don't I have a daddy? Why can't I meet my daddy? Why doesn't my daddy come to see me?'

How you answer these questions depends on whether or not you used an anonymous donor. Women who have arranged for the donor to be anonymous have made a decision for the child that can't necessarily be reversed. Some women have decided against anonymous donors in order to be able to tell the child who the biological father is. They felt more comfortable knowing they could at least tell the child his name. Other women have asked friends to be donors so that the child could have a close connection with his or her biological father.

Whether the donor is known or not, there are various ways to explain the situation to your child. To some women, it makes sense to differentiate clearly between donors/biological fathers and fathers/daddies. A man who donates sperm and has no parental responsibility for the child which results is merely a donor. He only becomes a father if he cares for the child in some important way and is a major presence in that child's everyday life. Thus, father-hood is defined as a social role. It does not automatically result from the biological act of donating sperm. Children may know their donor and have some kind of relationship with him but still not have a father. To give a man the status of father when his only contribution is a spoonful of sperm and ten minutes of his time seems to be making a fetish of fatherhood. To other women, this kind of separation between the concept of donor and that of father is too far removed from established concepts to be acceptable.

It is an exciting part of parenting to watch your child's growing awareness of the world and to see what they make of the place. While it is a challenge, it can also make you feel anxious and angry. You are bound to worry about difficult situations they could encounter at school or with friends, about hostility they might be exposed to that they are too young to understand. You might be apprehensive about the consequences of their innocent remarks. What will happen if they tell their teacher you're a lesbian or that they have no father? Many mothers of SI children have strongly felt the need for themselves and their children to meet and share experiences with other mothers and children.

One useful aid to telling children is to read them books which show children with lesbian mothers and which raise the issue of donor insemination. Seeing their kinds of family validated in print can have a positive impact on young children, not to mention on mothers. Although they have their faults, it is wonderful that these books are available and that there is beginning to be a choice. A number of children's books have appeared in the last few years, which are reviewed in Appendix A, 'Resources and Reading List'.

### ● Shaheen (1992)

*Since I had Anton, I've met a lot of lesbians who want to have children and who want the donor to be involved. It really made me think what I would do if Anton asks to see his daddy. He's at the stage where he is asking (he is 3), and as he gets older, he will ask more and more. I did think that if he does persist, I will get in touch with the woman who knows the donor and ask her if she will ask him whether he could be approached, and whether he would be interested in seeing Anton. But I would only do this if Anton persisted and seemed to be very upset and disturbed. I know the donor's name and where he lives. I have photographs of him, though they are not very good.*

*It took me a long time to get Anton to call me by my name, Shaheen. He knew me as mummy. I wanted him to know me not only as mummy but as a person in my own right, not just a mummy. First of all when I told him my name was Shaheen, like his name was Anton, he wouldn't have it. I was mummy and that was it. I think he thought that I was trying to tell him that I was someone else, but finally I drummed it into him. Recently, Anton asked me why I am brown when he is so white. I told him that it was because my dad was brown. He then asked where his daddy is. I said, 'You haven't got a daddy. You've got two mummies. Who are your two mummies?' He just laughed at me and said, 'Mummy and Shaheen.' I expected him to say Jackie and mummy but he didn't. To all intents and purposes, my former partner Jackie is his other mother. Maybe he thought I was pulling his leg.*

### ● Pat (1986)

*I told Dean (my 9-year-old son) what I was doing first of all and he was excited because he wanted a baby brother. If I say something to him, I ask him a little while later, to see if he got the message and he asks me more questions as it sinks in. He tends to* listen to you and say, 'Oh yeah, yeah, yeah!' and you don't know if it's sunk in or not. But he seemed to know what I was talking about. All he's known is me being a lesbian and he knows that men and women also have relationships and have babies. I tried to explain to him as best I could how I was going to get this baby! He seemed to think that was all right. He was quite excited when I got pregnant and he was glad he had a sister in the end. But the only thing that Dean didn't like was that Marcy was the same colour as me and he wanted her to be the same colour as himself, because he felt like there were 'two of you' and there was only 'one of me', plus it's a girl, so 'I'm the only one.' But now my lover's here and she's the same colour as he is, so it doesn't bother him at all now. That's the only thing.

I think you should explain to them, though, what people actually think about it. My mum never told me that I was any different from anybody else in terms of colour. Although you see yourself as different, you don't think it matters. It wasn't till I went to school that I found out how different I was.

It's good to say that there are two ways of conceiving, but you have to explain how other people are going to react, because otherwise he's going to come out with something and someone's going to put him down. Dean knows that if his friends are going to find out, they're probably going to say things and tell people in school. He had one friend that used to stay with us but I said to him maybe he shouldn't stay so much, because I'm not going to tell my lover to go home because his friend is staying, though I don't flaunt it at all. And the friend did say, 'Marcy's got two mums.' Dean got upset because he thought he was saying that I was a lesbian. We've spoken to Dean about it, and he says, 'I don't care what they say.' But we still have to say, 'We know you don't care but ...' They could really hurt him with it. People aren't as sensitive as you think they are – just because they're your friends doesn't mean they won't say anything bad. That is a bit of a cross to bear. But he knows what's what and he doesn't say things. I don't think he's too bothered. I think he has more trouble about his colour than anything else. I'll have to see what he's like when he gets older. I think it will matter more then.

Dean has got a father somewhere and I know where he is and he can find him if he wants to when he is older. But Marcy doesn't have that. I am going to tell her how she was conceived [through DI at BPAS – British Pregnancy Advisory Service]. At

*BPAS, they say to you, 'Would you tell your child when it gets older that it was through insemination that you conceived?' I got the impression they wanted me to say no. I felt that I was supposed to say, 'No, I'm going to tell her that I had a relationship with a man and that's how she came about.' [At BPAS, other women have said that they would tell the child that he or she was conceived through donor insemination, and that answer was accepted.]*

## ● Sheila (1986)

*The other day a mother of a child at Tim's school told me her son thought that Tim had no father. 'I told him he must have a father,' she said to me. When I said, 'No, he's right. Tim hasn't got a father. I had him on my own and he's never had a father,' she looked surprised. I told her I had wanted a child but I didn't want a man to be involved, so I decided to get pregnant and be a single mother from the start.*

*It is important to me that Tim has no father. Saying and thinking that we don't know who his father is, or that we don't know his father, doesn't describe my feelings about his conception. He never did have a father, as far as I'm concerned, and that seems much clearer and more positive to me. We sometimes talk about how I asked a man for some sperm to start him off. Tim asked the other day if the man who gave me the sperm to start him off was a nice man. I said I didn't know him but that I'm sure he is. He doesn't really understand yet that many people find our way of getting pregnant strange. Well, I've told him but I don't think it has sunk in. He knows lots of people don't like lesbians too, but I don't think he can really understand what that means until he has experienced it for himself. To a 6-year-old, the world is so full of new concepts and ideas that conception and pregnancy is just one of many. And having or not having a father is no more or less significant to him at the moment than having or not having a grandmother or cousin.*

*For me, as time goes on, the importance of conception fades into the dim and distant past. I can't even remember what the various donors looked like any more, or where they lived. Even from the beginning, Tim has been himself. Possible biological connections have never seemed very significant to me, but they get even less significant as Tim gets older.*

● *Jean (1991)*

The response of Alice (the daughter of my lover Cathy) to her family unit has been completely accepting. She's always been open about the fact that she has two mummies. She's been very lucky because she was born at a time when a number of our lesbian friends were also pregnant. She went to a childcare group when she was 2 where there were more lesbian mothers than straight parents. She knew a whole load of other kids in her peer group who were also children of lesbians or single parents. What we used to do was name all the children who lived differently, who didn't have fathers or who had fathers they never saw. They were the majority of her friends and that makes a really big difference. Even when she went to school, it didn't appear to be a problem. She has been supremely confident and assertive about it with other children. She never felt she had to hide it. She is a confident child in herself anyway, like first children often are. Her family unit hasn't been a problem.

When I go to her primary school, the children in her class all call out to her, 'Alice, Alice, here's your mummy.' Then always somebody says, 'Alice, Alice, have you got two mummies?' She says yes in a very matter-of-fact voice. Alice is lucky with her teacher, who is quite open and supportive. She read Heather Has Two Mommies to the class, and Alice was made to feel quite important and special because she did have two mummies. It has been a status symbol rather than an area to be teased about it.

Despite that, when she got to the age of about 4, she started to ask about her father. This was to do with having moved into a wider social network where fathers were more dominant than she had experienced when she was small. She used to demand to see him and to know his name. We only had one photograph of him in our album that a friend had given us. We told Alice that her father lives close and that he would be prepared to see her. She wanted to know why he didn't come to see her. Obviously that's what they will think. So we had to explain about the arrangement we made with him in order to make her. This was an arrangement to use his sperm because we wanted the baby. We told her that he was very kind and donated sperm but he didn't want to be a father. We said we didn't think that Alice needed a father and two mummies. She sort of accepted that but a bit sulkily. Having been told how a child is created biologically, she then felt hurt that the other person wasn't more interested in her. It was an emotional response to not having a father after understanding the mechanics of reproduction.

The trouble for us was that we knew the donor personally. We had this awful dilemma about whether to try and ask him to make contact with Alice and what that would mean for the rest of us. Finally, as a result of Alice's constant demands, Cathy and I arranged a meeting with him. He was sweet but he was very clear that he had arranged to be a donor in order for Cathy to get pregnant. He didn't want any parental involvement, but he had always said that he would talk to Alice and that he'd like to meet her. He wanted to meet her without us being around, which is actually a bit difficult for a young child to cope with, so we didn't feel great about that. When it was suggested to Alice that she meet him on her own, she didn't want to. By this time she was about 6. She had lost interest in him by then. There was a patch between the ages of 4½ and 5½ when she wanted to know all about her father. It's very interesting because this is just what my daughter, Elaine, is getting into now. It definitely goes with their age.

I'm very happy that we resolved it without Alice meeting the donor. I was very worried about it. I thought it was unnecessary and that we would be creating far more trouble than it was worth. It was easier for me to be more rational about it than Cathy, because Cathy felt so terribly guilty that she had deprived Alice of a father. She felt guilt that she hadn't given her child what she wanted. It's also complicated by the fact that it's impossible for my daughter, Elaine, to meet her father. If Alice was able to go off and meet her father and Elaine couldn't, it would cause another upheaval in our family unit.

When Elaine reached the age of 4½, she asked me about her father. It's been quite reassuring in a way to see that they both have the same responses. It's to do with their age and intellectual development. At that age, they are much more aware of social groupings. They want to know why they are different.

When Elaine asks me about her father, I tell her everything I know, which is only his first name. I don't know his surname. I have no photographs of him. My first reaction was to beat my breast with guilt. Oh God, why can't I give her the information that she needs! I kept thinking that I must contact him but something stops me because I know he doesn't want that. He got completely freaked out about what he'd done after Elaine was born, and changed his mind about having any contact with us.

*In a way, it's easier to deal with Elaine's questions because there is only so much I can tell her. She can get mad and say, 'It's not fair. I want to see him. Why doesn't he want to see me?' I just have to say the same things over and over again – that wasn't the arrangement. There are such clear boundaries around the whole area for Elaine that I think it's easier for her. Also from my experience with Alice, I hope this little blip of father-interest which comes between the ages of 4 and 5 will pass. On the other hand, it might be quite deep-seated with Elaine and it might carry on and on. Who knows! You can't predict.*

*Elaine has never been as accepting of having two mummies as Alice. She's always wanted a daddy. It's very different for Elaine, because the majority of her friends come from straight nuclear families and are boys. She's had a very different experience from Alice. It's partly because she's always played with a best friend who has a mummy and daddy. She's spent a lot of time around there with him. She's been exposed far more than Alice to the nuclear family set-up and is much clearer about what is different about us and, as she perceives it, what she hasn't got. Alice was never that interested in men, but Elaine has always wanted friendships with men and was very keen on men. I felt guilty that she always wanted men.*

*I think it's quite important that our kids have their own community. I think it makes them feel much more secure to know there are others like them. And that's what Elaine didn't have, because there weren't any other lesbians getting pregnant at the time I did that I knew. There was only one friend really. I didn't go to postnatal groups because I was so depressed after I had her. She hasn't got the same peer group as Alice. Now that she's old enough to play with them, she can slot in with Alice's peer group.*

*It was quite interesting when we went to visit a friend who has a son by self-insemination the same age as Alice [7]. There were Alice, Elaine and Rhys making paper chains. We overheard this conversation, which appeared in the middle of their playing and then receded again.*

*Elaine said to Rhys, 'Is John your daddy?'*

*Rhys said, 'No, no. He's not my daddy. I haven't got a daddy.'*

*Alice and Elaine both said in chorus, 'Oh yes you have.'*

*Rhys said, 'No, I haven't. I've got a birth father.'*

*Elaine said, 'Oh.'*

Rhys explained, 'A birth father is somebody who helped make me, but he's not a father who lives in my house with me.'

Alice said, 'Oh yeah. Just like us.'

Elaine said, 'Pass me the red paper.'

They were dealing with the issues of their own lives by themselves. Elaine was really lucky that she was sitting there with two kids who said that they hadn't got daddies and that they're all in the same situation.

### ● Laura (1992)

Communicating with my daughter about her conception by SI began the moment she was first in my arms. I think my friend Sheila and I must have talked about this before the babies were born, and we must have said it would be the first thing we would whisper to them. Writing this brings tears to my eyes, such a strong feeling that they would know, almost as well as they knew any aspect of their lives, almost as traditional tales are told, at mother's breast, knee ... and it is true I did whisper it to her, 'Once upon a time there was a woman who very much wanted to have a little baby like you. So she talked to some men she knew and asked them if they could give her some sperm. They agreed. So on this particular day, she went to their house and they gave her some sperm in a little glass jar, and she put it into her vagina. And the sperm swam up her vagina through her cervix, into her womb, and there it met an ovum coming down from her ovaries and the sperm and the ovum joined up together and you began to grow.'

Other times we've talked in the bath about insemination, lots. She's occasionally wanted to meet the donors, and last year we nearly did it, because some work I was doing brought me again into close contact with one of them. He's a nice chap, they all were, and we discussed meeting up. To him it was fine, with me it was fine, but in the end we didn't quite make it. He was under lots of pressure, and so were Jenny and I. It just wasn't feasible to go half-way across London on a Tuesday evening. I guess we'll have more luck one day soon, when our lives calm down enough.

### ● Mary (1986)

The basis of the agreement on which we did SI with the men was that we wouldn't talk to anybody about it. In fact I don't know who Owen's father is. The children have never asked directly. The subject of their coming into the world does come up from time to time. I talk to them about a group of gay men who all gave sperm. They're only 6 now and they've never said they've wanted to get in contact with any of those gay men. It is possible in the future that they may want to do that. It's difficult to say how I'd respond. When they're older, if they want to try and trace back contacts and get in touch with the men, that's up to them. I wouldn't stop them doing it.

Since the children were really tiny, even before they could understand words, I've talked to them about self-insemination. They just accept it as being part of their lives. It's not a problem at all for them to accept SI as a way of conceiving. But they also know very well about other people's homophobia and heterosexism, and they have to deal with it. I don't need to tell them, 'It may be better not to talk about this at school.' I've told them in general about lesbian issues – that they need to be aware that if they talk about this at school, some people don't agree with lesbians having children and might be quite shocked by what they say. But they take responsibility for dealing with specific things. They're forced into that position because everything around them is telling them that heterosexuality is the norm and is the only acceptable form for relationships.

● *Jill (1992)*

I decided early on that honesty with my son about his paternity was essential and the only possible option. He became interested in how babies are made etc. at the age of 3 and I knew it wouldn't take him long to wonder about his own situation. When he asked me, I told him that a nice man who I didn't know had given me some sperm because I wanted to have a baby on my own.

He accepted this and, at certain times in the intervening years (he is now almost 7), has had periods where he's frequently asked me why I didn't want him to have a dad and saying that he wished he had one. At first, the latter upset me a lot, but I've gradually got used to it and now realize that the dad he wants is an idealized figure who constantly buys him toys and plays endless games of cricket and football with him. Most importantly, I've tried to keep the lines of communication open between us, and to listen to his feelings and to answer his questions honestly. I'm prepared *for him to perhaps be angry with me when he's older, because he may feel that I deprived him of something precious, but I believe that, with the strong bond and good relationship that we have, we will get through it.*

● **Toni (1991)**

*Before my daughter, Claire, was born, I had thought vaguely about how I would explain self-insemination and the donor/father person to her, but my experience of actually telling her has taught me that telling is not a one-way process, nor is it a once-and-for-all-time matter.*

*I explained the procedure of self-insemination in very simple terms several times between the ages of 2 and 5. It was hard to say how much she took in, and I didn't want to overload her. I got a few right-on books on the subject, which were dreadfully tedious, and neither of us could be bothered to look at them more than once. She did become very interested in 'sexing' (having sex) when she was 5½, after a month-long visit by a boy her age who introduced her to some practical explorations of the subject. Since then, she has been much more curious. Recently she asked again how babies are made and I explained how she was conceived. It obviously sounded plausible and acceptable to her. I then went on to tell her about the other method in common usage. By the look on her face, I knew that comprehension had dawned. Disgusted, she reeled back in her chair and in a shocked, horrified voice, said, 'I don't like the sound of that at all.' I had to laugh and will stay tuned to the same channel to see what reaction she has as a teenager.*

*When Claire was just 3, she began to ask about her daddy. In fact, 'Where is my daddy?' were nearly her first words, after she had perfected the word 'No'. I gave her my prepared line that her daddy was a very nice man named Pierre who had generously given me sperm so that I could have a baby, and she was that very-much-wanted baby. I had decided not to describe him to her as a donor because I can't relate to that term. He was a real person, not just a source of sperm. In my mind it didn't seem very real to make a distinction between the donor and the daddy.*

*She bought this story for about a week. Then, out of the blue, came the next logical question. 'I want to see my daddy. Where is he?' Again I was ready with the line about different kinds of families with different kinds of daddies. We have the kind of family where the daddy does not live with us. Some families have two mummies and no daddy. Some have one mummy and one daddy where they all live together. In other families there is one mummy or only one daddy. Then again, there are daddies that live with their children all of the time, some of the time or hardly ever. Surprisingly, I was able to provide examples from people she knew for most of these variants of family life. I was quite pleased with myself. At the end of this recital, she said very firmly, 'Why can't I see my daddy?'*

*If I had never known Pierre, I suppose Claire's curiosity could have gone no further. But in fact I did know him (although I had had no contact with him since I became pregnant) and I was happy about them meeting. Since he had only agreed to be a donor, I didn't feel I had the right to change the conditions we had set years before. Unknown to me, Pierre was thinking along the same lines. He too wanted to meet Claire, but felt he couldn't invade my territory or presume that he had a right to see the child he had made possible. I wrote to him and he and I met without Claire to discuss what we were getting into.*

*I tried to be very casual when I told Claire, then age 4½, that she would meet her daddy for the first time, but she was absolutely manic when we finally did meet at a museum. She held his hand, told him she loved him and dragged him around the museum at a furious pace. She certainly had internalized a traditional view of 'daddy' because she tried to get me and Pierre to hold hands too as we walked along the street.*

*Pierre began coming over about once or twice a month, and we gradually evolved relationships which became very friendly and not so intense. Two and a half years on from that first meeting, Claire was relaxed about her daddy and happy with the friendship they had. She knew who her daddy was but seemed not to want anything more. It felt more comfortable to me as well to have Pierre's involvement with us, and to be able to tell Claire something more than that her daddy was a very nice man.*

*However, nothing stays the same. When she was 6½, Pierre started coming by once a week and the dynamics changed again. The quiet and peaceful play sessions that he and Claire had enjoyed turned into angry scenes, with Claire rejecting him and accusing him of disturbing her powers of concentration. One day she flounced out of the room in her usual dramatic style, declaring that*

*I loved Pierre as if he were my son and it was obvious that I loved him more than her. When I probed a little deeper into why she was so angry, she came out with, 'Anyway Pierre's not a real daddy. A real daddy sticks his penis in a woman and lives with her.' Silently thankful that I don't have to live with a 'real daddy' (it must be dreadfully uncomfortable), I did my best to hear her anger and accept what she was feeling. I can't make her feel the same way I do about it. Her perspective will always be different from mine. Since then I've overheard her saying quite happily that she has the kind of daddy who doesn't live with us.*

*I have explained about me being a lesbian but have been cautious about telling her too much about homophobia. She is easily upset and tends to blow things up out of all proportion. When she was 4, she heard Ann Winterton, the Tory MP, on the television going on about how wrong it is for lesbians to have children. Claire was terrified that she wouldn't be allowed to live with me any more since I'm a lesbian. I know that Claire does hear a lot of rubbish from her classmates, especially from the boys. They tend to lay down the law, saying things like girls aren't allowed to kiss girls and it's wrong for boys to kiss boys. Sometimes she does get thrown by these statements. She wouldn't kiss me for three months, until she told me what they had said and I could tell her not to listen to stupid little boys. Now she's nearly 7 and a bit clearer about these matters. When the boys said that a lesbian is half girl and half boy, the halves being the right and the left, she told them that they were just wrong. I find it hard to get a balance between preparing her for the homophobia she will continue to encounter and terrifying her with reality before she is ready to cope with it.*

● *Bronwen (1992)*

*My son, Rhys, has always learned, along with the facts of life, that there are two ways to get pregnant. The sperm either gets in the vagina by a penis or you put it there by some other method. So he knows that and accepts that as normal.*

*As soon as Rhys first asked any questions about his father, I explained very simply about a friend who gave sperm. He must have been about 2½. He was pretty fed up about it, especially because the nursery where he was going was giving him a heavy time, saying he must have a dad. I had told the nursery that Rhys* understood that his father was a friend but he didn't have a dad in the parenting sense of the word. I didn't tell them all the details. I would have liked them to respect that but they didn't. All the staff were informed but it was particularly the religious staff who kept pestering him about it, telling him everyone must have a daddy. So he got pressured about it at nursery but also he felt he wanted a dad.

You can only talk to children in that tiny golden moment when they are interested, asking questions and able to hear what you've got to say. Those moments are rare. You have to seize your chance and sometimes you fluff it. It's just like telling them about sex. You can't lecture them. You can't hammer on at them all the time, saying, 'You were conceived by a donor. Listen to me.' You can't silence them for ever by fluffing it, certainly not if you're willing to talk about it, but you can silence them for quite a while.

I think it's bound to happen that children have misunderstandings. Between the ages of 2½ and 3, it became apparent that Rhys had somehow internalized at a pre-verbal stage that the man who was my lover when I was pregnant, and in the early months of Rhys's life, was his dad. He didn't remember this man because he had left the country when Rhys was about a year old. Rhys had got a very early memory of him being around and then leaving. Then he got muddled up and thought his dad was dead because I had told him that my dad was dead. He forgot all the other conversations we'd had about who his father was.

One of the golden moments that I fluffed was the time he said with tears in his eyes, 'I wish I had a dad. Why didn't you give me a dad?' I felt terrible because I do regret not having structured into my life a second parent figure who lives with us and has regular involvement. I don't regret not giving him a dad. I don't think I'd be very good at being a mummy in a heterosexual relationship living with a daddy. But I still have ambivalent feelings about not having somebody that I am very close to living with us. If I had my chance again to respond to his question, I would have given him more space to be fed up and angry about it. What I did was to tell him very confidently that he has lots of people who love him dearly – David, the man who's very involved with him and is a close friend, my best friend, his grandma, his cousin. I tried to comfort him with the people he had against the person he felt he hadn't got, but in retrospect it came out a bit pathetically. I think he felt slightly silenced and went quiet and didn't complain about it for *another six months. Very occasionally, last thing at night or first thing in the morning, he'd say that he wished he had a dad. I wish I had given him more space to really feel his feelings and be cross about it. However, I'm sure that I'll have more of those chances.*

*He knows the donor as a friend who is the father of some friends of his who live in a different town. Rhys likes him and sometimes calls him his father but not his dad. He distinguishes father as somebody who gives the sperm, the biological father, and dad as being a social role when a man wants to live with you and look after you. These definitions were jointly worked out between me and the donor. I'm surprised that his children and Rhys don't talk to each other more about it, as they see each other two or three times a year. Rhys told them but they don't seem very interested in discussing it at the moment. The donor and his partner didn't want it to be a big deal. They wanted it to come up when it was appropriate.*

*Because I've had relationships with women and with men, and his close adult friends do as well, he doesn't distinguish between me having boyfriends or girlfriends. He's totally innocent that there should be any funny feelings about lesbians. I thought he should be prepared in case anybody says anything hurtful to him when he talks to other people about me having a girlfriend, so I did tell him that some people feel it's a bit funny to be lesbian or gay, and he looked completely uninterested and surprised and thought it was just one of those wrong things like racism. As far as I know, he hasn't come across any anti-lesbian prejudice. Because I don't have anybody living in an open lesbian relationship with me, my sexual relationships have not really impinged on his consciousness. He doesn't think it's funny at all. He doesn't make any issue over it.*

● *Kath (1986)*

*One of the commonest responses from heterosexuals mainly is what we're going to say if Ruth asks about the father. The answer is the truth. There's nothing else to say. She was totally chosen. He was somebody that didn't want to be a father. He felt that it was good that she should have two mums. That was one of the reasons he agreed to do it. If at some point she says she wants to meet him when it feels like it's reasonable to do that, then I guess we would backtrack as much as we could. I sometimes think maybe that information (about the donor's identity) should be deposited with somebody else. I just do not want to know.*

*It's going to be interesting. I have anxieties about how she's going to grow up, whether it will be harder having two mothers. In some ways, that's inconceivable as well. She's got two adults around, totally into her. There is no way that she is going to directly suffer from growing up in the situation she's in. It's brilliant. She has everything going for her. It's other people's reactions that could be damaging.*

*(1992)*

*Before Ruth was even conceived, we were clear that we would never tell her anything less than the truth about her genesis. Telling that truth has never been a problem. We can't remember exactly how she first broached the issue of 'how she came to be' and whether it arose from questions related to conception or fathers. We had already created a context by talking to her about the diversity of families, which was reflected in her own experience. At some point, she asked about having a father and we explained that there is more than one way to make a baby, and that she was made from an egg in Judy's tummy and a sperm, which had been given to us by a very good man who didn't want to be a daddy but thought we would make very good mummies and wanted to help us.*

*We are very careful to make the distinction between fathers and donors, which she understands and owns, to the point of asserting to a clumsy teacher who insisted that 'everyone had fathers' (meaning sperm), that she didn't have a father, and sol-icited our help in explaining the mechanics to her teacher. Her mates in the class, knowing that she has two mummies, confirmed her assertion. This was when she was 5. She has checked out the question once or twice and is always happy with the answer, and has never shown any interest in the donor figure. She has never seemed at all concerned about it.*

# A few words from the children

The people most affected by our decision to get pregnant are our children. Children are rarely listened to in our society, but what they have to say about their lives is valid. The issues that are important to them may not be the same as those of their mothers. Their voices need to be heard, especially by lesbians considering parenthood. In this section, I have interviewed a boy and a girl, both aged 12, who were conceived by self-insemination and have grown up with lesbian mothers. I chose them because they have each had twelve years of experience to draw on.

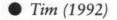 *Tim (1992)*

*Self-insemination is just about having a baby without having sex. What's the difference? The theory is that lesbian mothers and gay people are going to love their children much more because they have to try really hard to get their children. They must want it. They can't do it by mistake. I agree with that. I do really feel wanted and cared for.*

*I would say I'm a happy person. I got the Happiest Scout Award on the first scout camp I went to. They said that there were big arguments about who to give the different awards to, like the Most Adventurous Scout Award and the Most Helpful Scout Award. But when it came to the Happiest Scout Award, everyone agreed it should be me.*

*I like singing and I sing in a choir. I like quite energetic things like cycling and swimming. I don't like sports that much. I suspect that may be because of not having a dad. My mum has arthritis and she doesn't play any sports. Sometimes I do feel a bit different because even though I like watching football, I've never been to a football match. I'm quite disappointed about that. I'd quite like to see Arsenal play, but I suppose I can see it on telly. I have no desire to play football. Playing football is just boring to me.*

*I think a lot of my friends are rougher than me. Their fathers teach them to fight, which makes me very glad I haven't got a dad because I don't get into fights. If a kid is brought up to be tough, he'll go and smash someone's head in if he gets called a name. I'm definitely glad I don't have a dad to teach me that attitude. My mum does not agree with hitting anyone. If she sees anyone else hitting someone, she'll tell them off, which I think is good. However, I'm not the kind of person who can be picked on easily. I do defend myself and I am quite protective of my friends. I don't feel I'm a right softy. I'm just like any other kid. I don't let people bully me.*

*When teachers say something like, 'Get your dad to sign*

this', I either ignore that or I go up to the teacher and ask if they definitely mean dad or can I get my mum to sign it. Sometimes they definitely mean dad, like on sports days. The teachers who represent our colour would say, 'Go and get your dads and get them to join in the race for our colour.' That would be really embarrassing because I couldn't. I would either have to say I haven't got a dad or he's not here. That's how I tackled it. But I feel fine about it.

Sometimes I have to lie and sometimes I don't. When I go on holiday with Anna and her girlfriend, people I meet always find it confusing. I consider Anna part of my family, like another relation. I don't know what to call her. I don't know if it matters what I call her. She's almost like my dad really. First of all, they meet her and I say she's my mum because it's much easier. When they come into my tent to play cards or something and they see another woman, I just say one's my mum and the other's a friend from London. I've met some nice kids with horrible parents, and as soon as I see their parents I think it's not a good idea to tell them. I don't lie about it to anyone I know I'm going to be with for more than a couple of weeks. I would never lie to a schoolmate.

I have no desire to meet my father. I was saying the other day to Sheila (my mum) that when I'm 20 or so, I might like to track down my dad and meet him, but I don't really have a strong desire to find him. I'm slightly curious. It would be kind of interesting to find out who this person is. I would like to know his name. Sheila doesn't know much about him at all. If people ask me what my dad does, I just have to say I'm not quite sure. It sounds strange if I say I'm not sure. Sometimes I say I don't have a dad, but sometimes I say he's a lorry driver just to keep them happy.

Kids at school make these terrible jokes about gays and lesbians. This is one: 'There were two men in a bed feeling happy, so happy got out.' It is disgusting. I just don't find them funny. Kids think that gays and lesbians are people to make fun of, that they aren't as normal as their parents. They need to make fun of somebody. When I was in the fourth year junior, I went to the head teacher about these horrible jokes. I wanted him to come down hard on people who do this. But he is the kind of person who is very understanding, and you really feel that you are being listened to, and then he does sod all about it.

One day one of my best mates worked out that I wasn't finding the jokes funny. He asked me, 'What's the matter? Don't you find them funny?' That's when I told him that my mum is *lesbian. He went all embarrassed and said, 'Sorry about those jokes, Tim.' He was embarrassed that he had made fun of me. I could see that he didn't really want to hurt me. I had thought I was probably going to have a bad time of it, but actually it was a good reaction and I felt glad I had told him.*

*I think it is quite important to know other children of lesbians. I need to chat with somebody else about it. I think I need to know that I'm not the only person in the world like this. Sheila has started up a lesbian mothers' and children network. That's great. I feel more relaxed with those people because they will understand. I feel relaxed with people at school, but there is still always a little bit of a burden to carry in case anyone should mention something about my dad. I don't think any of my mates at school are from single-parent families, though I'm not sure. Maybe they are really from single-parent families and they just say their parents are divorced.*

*Last year, there was the big scandal about the virgin birth technique. We were listening to PM on Radio 4 while driving down the motorway. On the show, people were saying they thought it was selfish of the woman [to be single and use donor insemination]. It just makes me think how stupid those people must be. They were telling everyone to ring in if you had any comments on it, and when I got home, I rang in. I wasn't actually on the air. You have to leave a message on their answer machine. I said, 'I'm the son of a lesbian mum. She's single and she used the so-called virgin birth technique and I feel fine about it. I don't see anything wrong with it at all. It's certainly not selfish. In fact, I think I've got a better life than many kids.'*

*One of my mum's friends suggested that I ring up the local BBC TV station. So I did. I got put through to this woman who asked what I wanted to say. I told her what I'd said on PM and that I would like to go on TV, as my experience is relevant to what's happening and I'm upset about it and think it's disgusting what people are saying. She said, 'Can I speak to your mum? When would you be ready?' At this time, it was about 7 p.m. They arranged to come over to our house at 9 p.m. First of all they filmed us looking at my photo album of when I was a baby. There were all these pictures of Sheila holding me. They asked me questions like, 'Do you think your mum's being selfish? Do you think you would rather have a dad? Would you like to meet your dad?' There were lots of questions like that. It was really exciting.*

*They had a horrible priest or something on the show who kept saying, 'He's only an 11-year-old boy. When he's 22, I'm sure he'll have different views.' It made me angry. I felt like ringing him up and telling him that he doesn't know what he's talking about. Why can't he keep his nose out of it? He was saying that because I'm only 11, I can't have any views, that I'm not a proper person. I hate that kind of stuff. I'm very conscious of my rights.*

*It was on the next day. I told everyone that I was going on TV but I didn't tell them what it was about. Not many people watched it, because I don't think anyone believed that I was actually going on TV. Some of the teachers did watch it, and since then, they have reacted quite differently. I haven't heard, 'Give this to your mum and dad.' I hear more of 'Give this to your parents,' or 'Take this home.' I don't think I've heard any of the anti-gay jokes since. I've definitely raised the consciousness of my class-mates. I'm glad I told people, because it's got a lot off my back.*

*My mum has had three different lovers in my life. I was 6 or 7 when she got involved with the first one. I didn't find it hard at all. Sheila has good choice in lovers. I can usually trust her to bring home someone nice. It's a bit sad for the first week or so after they split up, but I can cope with it. I really don't mind that much. We don't see the first lover any more, but we still see the second one. She is really nice and so is the woman Sheila is lovers with now.*

*There are a lot of things that I like about my mum. She is really good in emergencies. She makes me have very healthy food. She doesn't let me have any of that Mr Whippie ice cream. I don't mind having healthy food occasionally, but not all the time. She will make me do jobs like washing-up and doing the bins. I do appreciate that, though sometimes I'd rather she didn't. She's into fairness.*

*A lot of boys don't cuddle their mums a lot. They wouldn't go in for a morning cuddle in their bed, or wouldn't want their mum to come into their room and give them a cuddle before they go to bed. I do. We're very close and I love my mum a lot.*

● *Jenny (1992)*

*I'll be 12 next week. I enjoy reading, especially science fic-tion but also old books. I do a lot of swimming. I play a baritone horn at school, which I really enjoy as well. Sometimes I go to the computer club and sometimes I go to a drama club after school. I* enjoy acting. I think I'd probably like to have something to do with the theatre when I am older. It will probably be designing, not actually acting. At school my favourite lessons are English and drama.

Both Laura and Tina are my mums. I don't think that there could be any difference in their relationships to me because they've always been my mums and they always will be. I love them both equally and very much. I can't remember when my mum and my mum split up. I was 3 or 4. I think I've blocked most of it from my mind. Now I live with my mum, Laura, in the week and go to school from her house. I go to my other mum, Tina, at weekends. I have to travel from south London to west London every Friday. I probably will start going on my own soon. Until a few months ago, we lived in west London and I went to school over there. I used to stay with Laura from Sundays to Wednesdays and with my other mum from Wednesday evenings until Saturdays. I did that for as long as I can remember. Because we just lived around the corner from each other, it was really easy. If my other mum moved here to south London, I'd like to go back to the arrangement we had before. I think that would be better, but this suits me fine. I've got used to it now.

My family includes other people too. In west London we lived in a communal house and have done for as long as I can remember. There were lots of women living there who I got really close to and who then moved out. It's often been difficult. When I was really little, I used to have a third mother. She wasn't a lesbian. She moved out when I was about 6 and moved in with her partner just around the corner. Now they've got two little girls who are my sisters, but she isn't really my mum any more.

There are several ex-lovers of both mums, some of whom are still in my family. Tina's present lover lives with my mum in west London. I see her every weekend and I get on with her quite well, though we do have our differences. I don't always feel completely OK with her. Tina is agoraphobic, so she is really dependent on people she trusts being there all the time. She can't go very far on her own. That makes me frustrated. I do feel protective of my mum.

Before that was Lotte, Tina's last lover. After my mum and my mum split up, the thing I first remember is Lotte coming. She was really nervous. She had bought me a massive packet of liquor-ice. I thought it was brilliant but Tina was cross with her for buying me liquorice. Tina wouldn't let me have any of it, but I just opened *the bag and immediately stuffed some in my mouth. When Tina and Lotte split up, it was very difficult because I was really close to Lotte. What really upset me was that Lotte was so upset. I was getting really worried about her because she wasn't eating. Now I see her a lot, at least every two weeks and often more. She lives near my school. I go to her house and I really enjoy seeing her.*

*At my first primary school, everyone knew that I had two mothers, though I don't know how. I was actually quite badly bullied there, but I don't think it had anything to do with having two mothers. I was just unlucky. At my second primary school, only my best friend knew and that was it. She was fine about it. At my secondary school, two very close friends know, but they're also both daughters of lesbians. They're in the second year and I'm in the measly first year, as they keep reminding me.*

*My second primary school was quite posh. The kids had rich parents and large houses and were mostly from the typical nuclear family, with brothers and sisters and a mum and a dad. I think I was a bit of an eye-opener for them – me being vegetarian and being green. After a while, by the fourth year, they were all vegetarian and green too. I don't know if that's got anything to do with having lesbian parents.*

*I think I've heard one anti-lesbian comment since I started secondary school. A friend came over when we were eating lunch and said, 'Oh God, we had this teacher. He's such a pervert.' I said to her, 'What does that mean? You can't say that. Just because somebody is different from you.' She kept saying, 'Yeah, but you know.' I kept saying, 'I know what?' She shut up after a while.*

*I have no father. I think I'm really better off without one. The girl next door is always arguing with her father, keeping me up till midnight. I've never felt that I've wanted a father and I don't ever think I will. I'd like to meet my donor at some point, but I'm not particularly desperate. It's not that important to me. He's not my 'father'. He's just my 'donor'. I know some women like their children to meet the donors, but I'm not bothered. I know enough about him. I know his name and roughly what he looks like. I know what his profession is. That's enough for me. I wouldn't track him down. It wouldn't be difficult to track him down because Laura still knows where he is.*

*Knowing other children of lesbian mothers has been very important to me. I think that if I hadn't had it, I would have felt quite isolated and lonely, shrunk inside myself and all on my own, but because I did have it, I don't feel bad. It has meant more contact with people and children like me. I suppose we're like our own little family within ourselves.*

*I don't think that having lesbian mothers has affected me. It hasn't given me any advantages. One disadvantage is that with all the lovers coming and going, and me getting close to someone, it hurts when they split up with my mums. But I don't think that that's made much of a difference.*

# Chapter six

# The Law

THERE have been major changes in the law in Britain in the last few years which are important for those of us doing self-insemination. The three laws which are most relevant are the Children Act 1989, the Human Fertilization and Embryology Act 1990 (HFEA for short) and the Child Support Act 1992. In this chapter I will explain how these Acts potentially affect us and what they say about the rights of the donor, the co-parent, the child and the mother, as well as the legal position of self-insemination itself.

## The legal position of self-insemination

There is no law against self-insemination in Britain, nor would it be possible to enforce such a law. At least one state (Victoria, Australia) has made unlicensed self-insemination a criminal offence punishable by a maximum of two years' imprisonment. However, in Britain, it is not a criminal act for a woman or a group to advertise for donors or for a magazine to carry advertisements for donors, nor is it unlawful for a woman to do self-insemination using fresh sperm on her own or with anyone's help.

The Human Fertilization and Embryology Act (HFEA) applies only to clinics offering donor insemination, not to self-insemination. HFEA is all about the licensing of 'treatment services' by the Licensing Authority, not about informal arrangements between women and men. Treatment services are defined as 'medical, surgical or obstetric services provided to the public or a section of the public for the purpose of assisting women to carry children'. A self-insemination group which screens donors and introduces them to interested women is not providing a medical service. However, it would be a different matter if a group took it upon itself to freeze semen. The Act prohibits the storage of gametes (eggs or sperm) without a licence. Storage in this Act means freezing.

Despite the homophobia that came out in the debate in Parliament, the HFEA does not prohibit clinics from accepting lesbians and single women. The guidelines to clinics published by the Licensing Authority are carefully worded to avoid discrimination against lesbians and single women and to make it possible for clinics to provide treatment to them. It is highly unlikely that the Authority or anyone else would take an interest in women doing self-insemination. (See Chapter 9, 'Donor Insemination Through Clinics'.)

## The legal position of the biological mother

The woman who gives birth to the child automatically has parental responsibility and never loses it unless she gives up her child for adoption. Even where the local authority takes the child into care, the mother keeps her parental responsibility, but in a limited way.

Parental responsibility is a new legal concept in the Children Act and means 'all the rights, duties, powers, responsibilities and authority which by law a parent has in relation to the child and his property'. Although she cannot lose her parental responsibility, she can share it with other people, who can acquire it by means of a court order. Each person with parental responsibility for the child can act independently of the other, but there are limits on the rights and powers of those who acquire it by court order (for example, they cannot change the child's surname or agree to the child being adopted). The one exception is the unmarried father (or donor), who gains equal rights with the mother when he has acquired parental responsibility through a court order.

## The legal position of the child

A child conceived by self-insemination is no longer considered illegitimate. There is no discrimination in British law against illegitimate children, and the concept has died a legal death. A child conceived by donor insemination in a clinic is legally fatherless if the mother is single. If the mother was married when she went for donor insemination, her husband is the child's legal father unless he did not consent to her 'treatment'.

In the Children Act, the child's welfare is the main concern of the court when any order is made to change the child's circumstances. There is a list of considerations (the 'Welfare Checklist') which must be taken into account by the court when deciding the child's best interests. In the Welfare Checklist, the court must consider:

1. the child's physical, emotional and educational needs;
2. the likely effect on the child of any change in circumstances;
3. how capable the person is of meeting the child's needs;
4. any harm the child has suffered or is at risk of suffering;
5. anything else about the child the court thinks is relevant.

The court must find out the child's wishes and feelings if the case is contested, and must take these into account when making any decisions, depending on the child's age and understanding. Children of 'sufficient understanding' may challenge decisions and can apply to be made a party to the proceedings. This gives a certain amount of power to the child to influence what happens.

## The legal position of the donor

If you go to a clinic for donor insemination, the donor is not the legal father of your child. Under HFEA, he abdicates his parental responsibility by signing a consent form. If you do self-insemination, the donor is considered an unmarried father, otherwise known as the 'putative father'. As such he has no legal rights, but he may acquire parental responsibility by applying for a court order under Section 4 of the Children Act. If the court grants him parental responsibility, he will share this with the biological mother and anyone else who has it. His responsibilities would be no greater than hers, but no less.

The donor is not automatically granted parental responsibility if he applies. The concept of parental responsibility and the presumption of both HFEA and the Children Act is not that the father has a right to the child but that a child needs a father. It is up to the donor to prove that he is the biological father by organizing genetic fingerprinting tests. If the test shows that he couldn't be the biological father, then he would not get parental responsibility under Section 4 of the Act (though he could reapply under a different section of the Act as a non-biological parent: see the section below, 'The legal position of the co-parent'). If he is the biological father, the court can act on its discretion, although the deciding factor must be the need of the child for a father. If the court decides the child would be better off with its father, it could grant parental responsibility regardless of whether the donor had ever seen the child, paid money for the child's upkeep or had his name on the birth certificate. Certainly it strengthens the donor's case in court if you do put his name on the birth certificate and let him establish a relationship with your child, but even without contact, the court is starting with the premise that the child should have a father.

According to the Welfare Checklist (see the section 'The legal position of the child'), the court is expected to consider how capable the donor would be of meeting the child's needs. Hopefully, the court would not give parental responsibility to a man who would be likely to harm a child in any way. Given the homophobia in the courts, it seems unlikely that a court would agree to a gay donor acquiring parental responsibility. However, it is not wise to assume that just because a donor is gay, he would not want parental responsibility, nor is it wise to assume the court wouldn't grant it to him.

As well as presuming that children need fathers, the Children Act also presumes that it is better not to make an order of parental responsibility rather than to make one. The court wants to be satisfied that giving parental responsibility will positively add to the child's welfare, not just meet the father's needs. In a situation where a child has been growing up quite happily with its lesbian mothers and has never had any contact with the donor, in theory the court could decide that giving parental responsibility to a complete stranger would not contribute to the child's welfare. In reality, it is probably safe to assume that most courts would be concerned about the welfare of a child growing up in a lesbian household and would decide to intervene in favour of the child having a father.

If the donor gets parental responsibility through a court order under the Children Act, he can potentially lose it if the mother or the child takes him back to court and complains. How this will work in practice remains to be seen.

Some women have arranged to co-parent with the donor and may welcome the clarity of the law on his position. Most women do self-insemination in order not to share parental responsibility with the child's biological father. The possibility of a donor acquiring parental responsibility equal to the mother's and more than that of a co-parent is very threatening. In the initial discussions, the donor may be genuinely uninterested in parenting. Usually that is the way it remains. Few men who donate sperm want to be active parents, and most have some decency about not going back on an agreement. However, anyone can have a change of mind. This is potentially more likely to happen if a donor has become involved with the child, but may also occur for other reasons.

How can women protect themselves from the risk of the donor acquiring parental responsibility? Using an anonymous donor is the most obvious way, but many woman want contact of some kind with the donor, at least to know who he is. A clear verbal agreement is a start. I have included a question in the 'Questionnaire for Donors' (Appendix C) asking if the man agrees that he would not claim parental responsibility for any child born from his donation. Drawing up an agreement may be another way. A verbal or written agreement would have no legal status, however. The Children Act prioritizes the needs of the child for a father and would not look kindly on a man waiving his right to claim parental responsibility. On the other hand, there is a small chance that it would be accepted as evidence of intent.

By law (in the Inheritance (Provision for Family and Dependants) Act 1976), a child has a right to make a claim to inherit from the donor's estate if he dies when the child is in need of financial support. The donor should be advised to make a will stating why he shouldn't make financial provision for this child.

You don't have to put the donor's name on the child's birth certificate; in fact you can only do this if the man agrees and signs the application form.

# Child Support Act

If you ever need to claim Income Support, the Child Support Act requires the father to pay child maintenance and requires you to name the father. This Act came into force in April 1993 and is part of the government's attempts to make fathers face up to their financial responsibilities. The Act is enforced by the Child Support Agency.

The Agency has issued guidelines saying that where a woman has 'made her own private arrangements for artificial insemination, the man concerned is the child's father and should be named'. The Agency will not accept the validity of any arrangements you might have made with the donor releasing him from parenting responsibilities. You are only exempt from naming the donor if you can show that 'there are reasons why harm or undue distress would result', or that you genuinely do not know who he is. The rule is retrospective, meaning it applies to women who did SI years ago. If you refuse to name the donor, you could have your benefit cut by 20 per cent (about £8.80 a week at 1993–94 rates) for the first six months, and by a lesser amount for another twelve months.

These guidelines do not apply to women who have had donor insemination with an anonymous donor at a clinic. In that situation, the child is considered to have no legal father. However, you will be asked for evidence that you did have donor insemination at a clinic.

These guidelines could discourage men from becoming donors and may persuade some women to have anonymous donors when they might wish to have a known donor.

# The legal position of the co-parent

The Children Act makes it possible for non-parents to acquire parental responsibility by applying for a court order under Section 8 of the Act. Under this section, grandparents, step-parents, aunts and uncles, guardians, friends, and presumably lesbian co-parents can be granted parental responsibility to share with the biological mother and anyone else who already has it. If the biological mother and the co-parent are living together and raising children together, it is natural to want to have some legal recognition of the co-parent's position. In theory, parental responsibility via a residence order would give the co-parent status with doctors, schools, officials of all kinds, and society in general. It could also be important for the child to grow up with parents of equal legal status and potentially equal power.

However, as long as everything is going well in their family life, it is not wise to risk coming to the attention of the authorities. It is the courts who interpret the law, and courts are predominantly homophobic. Regardless of what the law says, the courts are not favourably disposed to lesbians who are biological mothers, let alone to lesbian co-parents. The best advice at the moment is to stay out of the courts if at all possible.

The worst possible scenario is if a lesbian co-parent or a homophobic grandparent applies for a residence order and, while going through the Welfare Checklist, the court thinks that the child has already suffered significant harm or is likely to. Harm is defined in the Act as including damage to the child's intellectual, emotional, social or behavioural development, as well as their health. It is not hard to imagine a court worrying about the child's social development growing up with two lesbians, especially if the mothers are not middle-class or if any alcohol or drug abuse, mental illness or involvement with the police is discovered. The court can make an interim care order, taking the child into care for eight weeks or requiring supervision at home. While this scenario is very unlikely, it is not unimaginable.

The more painful situation arises where a lesbian couple splits up, and the co-parent wants to continue to have contact or to parent against the biological mother's wishes, or vice versa. The co-parent's legal position is very weak. Theoretically, she can apply for a residence order (Children Act 1989, Section 8 orders) which gives her parental responsibility as long as the order is in force. In theory, a separating couple could apply for a joint residence order. Anyone else who has gained parental responsibility, such as the donor or a grandparent, will be notified by the court and can object. Parental responsibility gained through a court order can be lost if anyone else with parental responsibility, or the child, takes it back to court. As mentioned before, the Children Act says that it is better not to make an order of parental responsibility rather than to make one.

'Residence' is the new term for care and control. A non-parent can automatically apply for a residence order if she has lived with the child for three years. Otherwise, she can apply with the written consent of those who have parental responsibility. The order lasts until the child is 16. She may request joint residence or sole residence, in which case the child would live with her.

'Contact' is the new term for access. The Act sees this as the child's right. The court would decide whether they think it is in the child's best welfare to continue seeing the co-parent.

The situation is painful, not just because of how the court might react to the conflict but because of what it says about the mother's acceptance of her partner's co-parenting, and because of how it might affect the children. Some biological mothers are not really prepared to share parental responsibility with a partner and will use any advantage, such as class or money, to deny their partner's claim. Equally, some co-parents may get away with abdicating their parental responsibilities against the mother's wishes because they have no legal position to hook them in. Ideally there should be a neutral conciliation service within the lesbian community to sort out these conflicts, without having to resort to the courts and the Children Act.

## When a mother dies

If the biological mother dies, the co-parent can potentially acquire parental responsibility in two ways:

1. If the mother has appointed her to be the child's guardian (Sections 5 and 6 of the Children Act). Appointing a guardian can be done by writing a simple statement, dating it and signing it in front of two witnesses. You do not need to go to a solicitor. A biological mother can also appoint someone to be her child's guardian by including it in her will or by making a formal deed.

2. By applying for a residence order. Especially if she has been living with the child and no one is contesting her application, she will have a good chance of getting parental responsibility. According to the Welfare Checklist, the court would rather not change a child's circumstances unless it is absolutely necessary.

Guardianship takes effect as long as there is no one else alive with parental responsibility. In other words, if the child's father had been married to the mother (even if later divorced), or he was an unmarried father who had acquired parental responsibility under Section 4 of the Children Act, the care of the child will automatically go to him. The only way you can get over this is if the biological mother has a residence order in her favour before she dies. This means that a court will already have decided that the child is better off living with her than with the father. However, this won't automatically prevent the father getting care of the child. In this situation all the co-parent can do is apply for a residence order when the mother dies. It will be very important that the biological mother has appointed her as guardian so that the court is aware of her wishes. If there is no father with parental responsibility, the co-parent will then automatically become guardian, with the full rights of a parent. If the mother has not named anyone to be the child's guardian, there will be a court hearing to appoint a guardian. Grandparents or others may step in at this stage and apply to become the guardian, or for a residence order if they want the child to live with them.

If the co-parent doesn't have parental responsibility through guardianship or a residence order, she can continue to look after the child informally. But she doesn't have any legal standing. She is considered to be a private foster mother and should really notify the local authority of what she is doing. The local authority has the duty to supervise private fostering arrangements and the power to disqualify or prohibit a person from privately fostering a child. If disqualified, you can appeal to a magistrate's court, but the court does not have to go through the Welfare Checklist. People have been disqualified because they have a history of very minor offences. It is a criminal offence, punishable by up to six months in prison, to foster privately if you have been prohibited. Because of this, it is a good idea for the biological mother to appoint the co-parent as guardian, or for the co-parent to apply for a residence order when the mother dies.

The co-parent should also make a will, whether or not she has parental responsibility, to make financial provision for the child in case she dies.

# Chapter seven

# *When SI Isn't Working*

GETTING pregnant may take a long time. Conception is not a mechanical process which must automatically work if all the conditions are right. Even if it appears that both the donor and the woman are fertile and the inseminations are accurately timed, it may take many months or even years of trying before success, or it may not work at all. It is sometimes possible to identify the reasons for not conceiving and occasionally to do something about them, but there is a great deal of unpredictability around conception. It is a process that is not within our control. The irony of the situation is that self-insemination is essentially a means of taking control of your life and choosing to become a parent against opposition; yet you cannot choose to conceive. This is hard for most of us to come to terms with.

Perhaps because of the lengths many heterosexual women go to in order to prevent unplanned pregnancies, we have the expectation that women can get pregnant whenever they want. It is true that there are women who conceive while using contraceptives or the first time they inseminate. It is not true that most women will conceive that easily. When you think of how complicated the female and male reproductive systems are and what must happen before a pregnancy results, it's more surprising that women get pregnant at all.

How long should you expect it to take to conceive? Certainly it is possible to conceive the first time, but there is no guarantee that this will happen. As far as I know, there are no statistics for the success rate of self-insemination (compared to donor insemination from a clinic). There is no reason to assume it will either be any quicker or take any longer than for women trying to conceive with male partners by sexual intercourse. Among heterosexual couples who try to get pregnant, one in ten are unable to conceive after one year of regular trying. In clinics using frozen sperm, which leads to lower pregnancy rates than fresh sperm, about one-fifth of the women who do conceive do so in the first month, and three-quarters in the first six months. The remaining quarter conceive between six months and twelve months. Although it is frustrating, there is no reason to worry about your fertility or the donor's until you have tried for at least twelve menstrual cycles.

# What affects fertility?

## Age

As you get older, it takes longer to conceive. Your fertility finally ends at the menopause, which usually occurs sometime between the ages of 45 and 55. From information collected by the Human Fertilization and Embryology Authority for a five-month period in 1991 (quoted in their second annual report, 1993), younger women were more successful with donor insemination at clinics than older women. The pregnancy rate per cycle was:

| | |
|---|---|
| Under 25 years | 10% |
| Aged 25–39 | 7% |
| Aged 40–44 | 3% |

The biological time clock is ticking away for each of us, but every individual is unique. What matters is not only your age but your state of health and whether you are ovulating. Some women do conceive while they are going through the menopause and many women are getting pregnant in their late thirties and early forties. If you are older, you might need to expect to try for longer before you conceive. Start off optimistically and don't worry if you are still trying after eighteen months.

## Miscarriage

About one in five recognized pregnancies ends in miscarriage, and some estimates give a figure of one in two of all pregnancies, most of which occur so early the woman may not even be aware she was pregnant. The majority of miscarriages occur in the first trimester of pregnancy. As you get older, your chance of miscarriage increases. Information from donor insemination clinics in Britain is that the rate of live births in older women is less than in younger women (HFEA, 'Second Annual Report', July 1993, p. 22). The live birth rates in 1991 by age were:

| | |
|---|---|
| Under 25 years | 8.0% |
| Aged 25–34 | 5.5% |
| Aged 35–39 | 4.0% |
| Aged 40–44 | 1.2% |
| Aged 45 and over | 0 |

### Infertility

Unfortunately, self-insemination does not guarantee a baby to everyone who uses it. Although it is not something to dwell on while you are trying to get pregnant, for some women there comes a time when you have to stop and re-evaluate whether it is worth it to you to continue. At the back of your mind, remain aware that it may not work.

# Fertility problems

Before you begin to worry about your fertility, first of all satisfy yourself that the donor is fertile. It is much easier to investigate infertility in a man than in a woman. Ask him to have a semen analysis if he hasn't done so already. Secondly, are you sure that you are inseminating during your fertile days? It is not necessary to focus on finding the day of ovulation, as this tends to cause too much anxiety, which you certainly don't need if you are having trouble already getting pregnant. But do you feel confident that you know roughly when you are fertile, by one of the signs mentioned in Chapter 3, 'Getting Pregnant'? This may be a time to use an ovulation kit for one or two cycles. Thirdly, are you having enough inseminations? Do not be surprised that you are not pregnant after a year of trying if you have only had one insemination each cycle.

If you are inseminating frequently, and are reasonably confident of the timing of the inseminations and of your donor's fertility, you may begin to question your own fertility. When should you worry enough about your fertility to consider seeking infertility investigations?

1. When you have inseminated during your fertile days with a fertile donor for more than twelve to eighteen cycles without conceiving.
2. When you do not menstruate.
3. When you have no fertile mucus at all.
4. When there are fewer than ten days between your temperature rise and your next period.
5. When you have no temperature rise during the cycle or very irregular cycles.
6. When you have miscarried more than three times.
7. When you know that you have a history of one of the following that could affect your fertility: anorexia; ovarian cysts; endometriosis; excessive exercise at the level reached by women athletes in training; recent use of the contraceptive pill or the injectable contraceptive Depo Provera; pelvic surgery; pelvic inflammatory disease; gonorrhoea; fibroids; ruptured appendix; internal bleeding into the abdomen or pelvis, especially if it was not diagnosed and treated early enough or has been chronic or recurring; infection as a result of childbirth, abortion or use of the coil.

If any of these applies to you, don't jump to the conclusion that you are infertile. But if you are concerned about your fertility, your GP can carry out some investigations or can refer you to an infertility clinic. Infertility services are patchy on the NHS, with great inconsistencies between health authorities, long waits (up to five years) and different definitions of who is eligible. You might not be seen until you have been trying without success for at least a year, while some say two or more years. At least 90 per cent of people seeking infertility treatment go privately. The British Fertility Society recommends that clinics restrict their infertility treatment to heterosexual couples in stable relationships. If the donor is willing, consider taking him along as your 'partner'. This will help you gain acceptance at a clinic, and will be useful in finding out if you are both fertile but not with each other. A man may have sperm which are incompatible with a particular woman's fertile mucus. During the fertility investigations, this could be determined by a 'postcoital test'. A sample of the woman's mucus is examined under the microscope shortly after insemination. The sperm will not be moving the way they normally do. In a clinic, this problem can sometimes be overcome by inserting the semen directly into the uterus, thus avoiding the mucus. This is not something women can do themselves. For women doing self-insemination or where the donor won't get involved with fertility investigations, it is best to find another donor.

For help finding a fertility clinic or for more information about infertility and its causes and treatments, contact Women's Health (see Appendix A).

# Trying to get pregnant: the feelings

If you have been doing self-insemination for a long time, don't underestimate the effect this can have on you. It is inevitable that the longer it takes to conceive, the more stressful it becomes. No matter how hard you may try to be relaxed and patient, you are likely to suffer extreme disappointment every time another period starts. It is a very emotional time and feelings of anger, frustration, jealousy, despair and inadequacy are not uncommon.

## Bereavement

The feelings women experience when not conceiving are those of bereavement. They go through the same stages of grief felt by those grieving over the death of an adult or a child. These stages are anger, denial and numbness. The grief is for the loss of potential – the potential child as well as your image of yourself as a mother. The bereavement is especially difficult because it is unfocused. There is no object to fix on – no memories, no clothes, no photographs. Until you stop inseminating, the grief is complicated by the hope that next month it will work. Only when you decide to stop inseminating can you work through the process of bereavement.

## Waiting

Waiting is a constant feature of the process of trying to get pregnant. There is the waiting while finding a donor, the two-week wait between the inseminations and the next period, the wait for fertile days and the next inseminations, the wait for referral to a fertility clinic, the wait for test results, the wait while you try some new method or drug suggested by the fertility clinic. Waiting can feel interminable and unbearable. It is usually thought of as time wasted doing nothing, yet at the same time you may feel unable to do anything else. The waiting fills the time.

## Jealousy and alienation

As soon as you want to be pregnant, you tend to notice pregnant women and women with children more than you ever had before. At first this is exciting, and you wonder what your child will be like when it reaches the age of the child you see. Eventually it becomes too painful. You may find yourself feeling alienated from your friends who already have children. It can seem as if everyone else is getting pregnant except you, and that people you know are caught up in family life while you are left on the outside. Intense feelings of jealousy and wanting to withdraw are not unusual. Those friends with children who are sensitive to what you are going through often do not know what is best to do. They may try to protect you by keeping their children out of your sight, but this may result in greater feelings of isolation and alienation as you share less and less with them. Or they may bring their children with them and risk intensifying your distress. Many people are so caught up in their own lives that they are unable to be aware of what you might be feeling. Trying to get pregnant is an invisible activity.

## Preoccupation

The desire to be pregnant and the practice of self-insemination can dominate your life. You can become preoccupied by your bodily processes and think of nothing else. You may feel betrayed by your body and angry that it is not doing what you want it to do. Just wanting to be pregnant can change how you view yourself and may exacerbate your desire for a baby. You may start out feeling enthusiastic but fairly detached, and yet find as the months or years go by that you become almost driven. Some people may label you as obsessive if you pursue infertility investigations or carry on for many years.

## Anxiety

Years of unsuccessful self-insemination inevitably create anxiety, especially if the wish for pregnancy becomes overwhelmingly important. You may worry about the method itself, the fertility of the donor, your own fertility, even whether you have a right to be a mother. You may be anxious about having sex after inseminating, even though sex does not cause miscarriage. You are likely to feel anxious about being turned down for fertility investigations because of not having a male partner. Women doing self-insemination often feel that they have to renew the decision to get pregnant every month. This in itself can be stressful.

# Coping strategies

There is probably no way that months and years of unsuccessful self-insemination can be made enjoyable, but there are strategies you can develop to protect your mental health while you are in the midst of it. From discussions with women doing self-insemination, I have compiled a list of suggestions.

## Acknowledge your feelings

Start by recognizing whatever feelings you are experiencing, even those 'unacceptable' feelings of anger, jealousy and despair. It is not necessary to do anything about these feelings but accept that you have them. Acceptance is not the same as abandoning yourself to them which can only lead to bitterness. Acceptance is about noticing what you feel in each moment, seeing it for what it is, and letting it go. Above all, be gentle and loving with yourself.

## Avoid blaming yourself

There is controversy about whether stress causes infertility, and you will probably hear this expounded as fact from one source or another. It is possible that stress does play some part, though it is difficult to prove such a statement. Unfortunately, you may interpret this to mean that somehow it is your fault you are not conceiving. This kind of thinking will not help. Whether or not stress causes infertility, it is definitely true that infertility causes stress, and stress is very hard to avoid. The advice to relax and avoid stress can be infuriating. It is not so easy just to forget about getting pregnant when you have to go to such lengths to organize the inseminations in the first place.

## Support

Long-term self-insemination is very stressful, and the women I talked to felt they needed as much support as they could get. It is usually helpful to know someone else who is doing self-insemination at the same time you are. There are a few SI support groups in existence, but if there isn't one near you and you would like to be in contact with women in a similar situation, you can try to set one up. If you are the partner of the woman inseminating, think about your own support network. Your needs are somewhat different and you may find the best support from other partners.

### Involve partner or friend

Suggestions that worked for some women were to keep your fertility awareness chart (see Appendix D) in a prominent place for both of you to consult, and to delegate responsibility for making arrangements and picking up the semen.

### Friends

Consider which friends you feel too vulnerable to expose yourself to. Protect yourself by not telling everyone. You don't have to tell people who are likely to be judgemental or dismissive. Make sure your friends know that you will tell them when you are pregnant. Although you know that they mean well when they ask, it can be too discouraging to be constantly reminded of your lack of success. Some women commented on the importance of keeping up friendships with women who are not involved with children, so you can get away from it all.

### Take breaks

If it is getting too much for you, miss a few cycles. You don't have to inseminate every month.

### Keep it all in balance

Don't worry about having the odd drink or cigarette. Stay in touch with your reasons for wanting a child in the first place. You can forget that the goal isn't to get pregnant but to have a child.

Weigh up the effect of the stress of not getting pregnant on your mental wellbeing against your desire to be pregnant.

# Reactions to miscarriage

Miscarriages are common and are a real bereavement. A miscarriage may bring up intense feelings of grief, anger, jealousy, guilt and anxiety. The grief may be as great when the pregnancy is at eight weeks as at eight months, though it is usually deeper the further along in pregnancy you are. You will need plenty of time to mourn. Some women find that their sense of loss increases after the miscarriage until the due date, and comes back on anniversaries in later years. Certainly it is a good idea for psychological as well as for physical reasons to wait until you have come to terms with the miscarriage before attempting another pregnancy. It is not uncommon to feel anxiety about the next pregnancy and, if or when you do conceive again, to hold yourself back from getting excited.

Many women do not tell anyone they are pregnant until the time of the greatest risk of miscarriage is past (at the end of the first three months). The danger with this strategy is that you risk isolating yourself with your grief, and you could lose the support you might otherwise have had if friends had been sharing your excitement and the reality of your pregnancy all along. However, people are not always as sympathetic as you might like. They often make insensitive remarks along the lines of, 'It's all for the best. There was probably something wrong with the baby anyway', or 'Never mind, you can have another.' People do not always know how to react to a miscarriage, because it isn't as real to them as to you, even if you have told them.

With a first miscarriage, satisfaction that you are able to conceive may accompany the grief. It is clear evidence that you are fertile and have every chance of conceiving again and carrying the baby to term.

● *Iona (1991)*

*The experience of defining and 'coming out' with my wish to have a child has been a several-years-long process, involving many changes and stages of confidence and vulnerability. I'm now 35½.*

On my 33rd birthday, I began to tell friends that I intended to go ahead and find a donor in order to self-inseminate. Two non-starters and much discussion, hope and anxiety later, I feel close to becoming pregnant – I may even be pregnant! Rose, my partner, and I have found, via another friend who was aiming to have a child, a donor with whom we're happy and who is committed and conscientious in helping us.

My life has taken many turns in the course of this search and often I've had to deal with a sense of time running out. However, the most overwhelming emotion of this process has been anxiety. Friends warned me of the impending and inevitable stress of self-insemination, which I took as seriously as one can in preparing for the unknown. I found that no event in my life has affected me at such a core level and in such a raw way. Perhaps this major upheaval, this churning of my senses, is a preparation for the greater changes ahead – certainly, two insemination cycles later, I have a certain perspective which enables me to see the turmoil as yet another part of the process.

One very odd sensation that recurred uneasily, until I learned to identify and communicate it, was that of being the centre of attention and of having many strings to pull. Suddenly those resources I'd sought – a loving and helpful partner, a committed donor, two flexible and supportive drivers, interested friends – represented almost unmanageable demands which I struggled to meet. A sense of isolation crept in, which I would imagine is very close to the desolation of motherhood on occasions.

My personal resources – energy, direction, motivation – became increasingly obscured by waves of anxiety and almost relentless anger that usually took hold of any warm feelings between Rose and me and tossed them into confusion, negativity and hurt. She had listened, supported me and gradually, over the years, identified her own readiness to participate in this process. Now, with reality drawing near, we were overwhelmed by a spiral of anger and fear.

Gradually, we found some space in the middle to talk and contact each other again, to voice fears and share plans and ideas. We looked at our individual needs and paid attention to each other's. I took up Tai Chi and worked less. As the pattern of inseminations became more familiar to all concerned, the sharing of responsibilities and need for delegation, the condensing of time and energy spent collecting the sperm, the need for a quieter social life, the dealing with grief and new beginnings, and the reality of lack of control all *became more obvious facets of a highly complex and challenging process.*

*This process will go on challenging us because it's about constant change. And we've begun now to accept that constancy of insecurity as part of real life. At heart, it **is** our real lives.*

### ● Rose (1992)

*For me, finding a donor has been more stressful than inseminating. Iona has only inseminated three times. It took quite a long time to find a donor. We both asked gay men who were friends of ours, but they didn't get back to us with their answers. They said they would, but we didn't know for ages if they were going to say yes or no. Finally we contacted them and asked if they wanted more time to think about it, which they said they did. After about six months, we asked them again and they finally said no, but they had actually made the decision five months before. They hadn't felt able to say even though we were giving them plenty of opportunities. It was frustrating and I feel really angry.*

*Since Iona has started inseminating with a donor we both really like, I quite welcome the fact that it might take another six months. Then I can get used to the reality of it. Last month, Iona was pregnant and miscarried and that was quite hard. Even though her period was late and then later, neither of us dared to say to each other that she must be pregnant. I was very casual, saying, 'It's been 39 days. How long was your longest cycle? Only 32 days. That must be something then.' That's how we were dealing with it. Then when she miscarried, I was very sad. It felt unfair. I was surprised at how disappointed I felt. That made me realize how much hope I actually had. In a way that is quite comforting, because it was a measure of how much I felt about it and how involved I felt in it all. I also felt amazed that it had happened so quickly. It was reassuring that she could get pregnant.*

### ● Kim (1986)

*My friend and I decided that we would like to have children, and, as I am the older of us, we decided that I would bear the first child and we'd see what we wanted to do after that. Once the decision was made, I began trying to become pregnant. That was mid-1978, and I gave birth to our daughter at the end of 1983. There* is many a tale to tell of those intervening years, but what is relevant here is that it took a long time.

Like most women I was brought up thinking that I would bear children. If I wanted children, then I would have them. I assumed fertility, and easy fertility at that. The emphasis in our lives was to prevent conception, and heterosexual women have to spend a lot of time and energy doing this, and have to place their health at risk in the process. It was disappointing and disheartening. Others in the self-insemination group were pregnant, so it seemed that I was the failure. I was so in tune with my body during these months of taking daily temperatures, checking mucus and feeling every minute ache and pain, yet I could not control it. I had no control.

It seemed I could not choose to become pregnant. It was frustrating not being able to make pregnancy happen, but, more than frustration, my body was causing me to feel a deep sense of failure in a way that I had not felt before.

After twelve months it was found, by chance, that I had a double uterus and that this might affect my fertility, but not to any great extent. There seem to be more reasons which cannot be explained by medical science for my not becoming pregnant during those months. Over the last few years, medical science has provided some answers to why women don't conceive, but of course, they don't know it all. And besides, lesbians do not have easy access to medical science! With self-insemination you feel you have a time limit, you can't just 'keep trying'. Self-insemination is often difficult to organize, it involves you with men and it takes over your life for a while. So it in itself can feel like a pressure.

This is not to be a tale of woe. It has the ending we wanted. We now have two children. We each have given birth to a child and they are lovely. But I want to help other women not to assume fertility. And also, when we think about having children, we should think about the possibility of having a disabled child. Hopefully if our lives aren't built on myths, we will have more control over them.

● *Mary (1986)*

I always thought that I would conceive without much problem. In the end it took six months. It was a very, very depressing experience altogether. It just seemed to take forever between ovulating, doing self-insemination and waiting till my period came. Waiting for two weeks was not enough time to forget about it but was a long time to be continually thinking about it. When I finally started bleeding, I would be really depressed. I used to take my temperature several times a day and read the same pages in books about pregnancy over and over again. Six months to be focused almost exclusively on trying to become pregnant seemed like an eternity. Yet, of course, six months isn't that long in terms of how long it takes many women to conceive. I think it is an incredibly difficult period.

It's also very different for a lesbian from the way it is for a woman in a heterosexual relationship. As a lesbian doing self-insemination you're making a very conscious choice, anew, every single month. Pregnancy never 'just happens'. There was a huge gap between myself and the heterosexual women with children I worked with.

My lover was already pregnant by the time I started. She was quite preoccupied with her own pregnancy but she did give me a lot of support, though it never seemed like enough. I was very pleased that she was pregnant. I never had any doubt about that. I was just incredibly frustrated about not being pregnant myself. Apart from her and the self-insemination group, which was fantastically supportive, there was nobody I felt I could talk to. I did feel very lonely and isolated.

## ● Jean (1986)

It was truly awful what my not succeeding at self-insemination did to us. It put an enormous strain on our relationship that was still shuddering from the impact of having a new baby in our lives [her lover Cathy's baby]. In retrospect, it is quite clear that I started to try and get pregnant when the baby was far too young. She was only eight months old. But my urge to get pregnant was such a strange and selfish one. I felt I'd supported Cathy through her pregnancy, labour, birth and the early months and now it was my turn.

The practicalities of organizing inseminations with a young child around were very difficult. There were problems with the availability of the donor when I needed him, and for month after month, it just did not work. I would inseminate – never quite at the right time and often only once a month – and then would come the tense two-week wait for my period. I would confuse the signs of premenstrual tension with early pregnancy, pore over Gordon Bourne [author of a popular book on pregnancy] and be absolutely *hell to live with. When my period was a few days late, which often happened, I would start to feel secretly elated, and then, at the first sight of those first drops of blood, would come a crushing depression. Finally, I got so depressed and things between me and Cathy were getting so bad that I took a two-month break from the whole process. My personality stabilized again – no more terrible mood swings at the end of my cycle – and Cathy and I had time to talk and plan things out before I started to try again.*

## ● Andrea (1991)

*Four years ago, my partner and I joined a group of women who were interested in, or already starting to try, self-insemination. Someone had a copy of the first edition of* Getting Pregnant Our Own Way, *and we were all so excited to find that not only were there other women to talk to about what we were planning, but someone had actually written about how to do it. We all bought a copy. I read mine from cover to cover, re-read it, kept it by my bed and read it on the bus. All of it, that is, except the bits written by women who didn't get pregnant. Superstitiously, I thought that if I read about them, then my chances of conceiving would be smaller, and anyway, I was excited, optimistic, curious, nervous; I didn't want to read about failure and disappointment. It would be like having the hangover while you were still tipsy.*

*But here I am all the same, having failed and been disappointed, having grieved and battled and refused to give up, and failed again and again and again. No baby to show for all that effort. No reward, no just deserts, no child of my womb. No new status, no joining in with the others, no belonging.*

*My hangover lasted for a very long time, although I know that many other women's have been longer. I tried to conceive for over three years, self-inseminating, using donors I knew or had at least met. By the time my partner and I had met, I had already decided that I wanted a baby, and I chose the first donor. My partner disliked and distrusted him; it was a disaster, the first real conflict in our relationship and a fundamental test of our love and loyalty. I felt that, by saying that she didn't want to use him and with no other donor on the horizon, she was trying to take my baby away from me. A timely holiday in Crete provided us with respite and a compromise: to approach an acquaintance, already a donor. He and his wife happily agreed and we embarked on the monthly ritual of counting, measuring, calculating, a two-hundred-mile round trip, sleeping on their floor and taking days off work, waiting, downfall.*

*I don't think that anyone else except other lesbians in the same position really can understand what this does to you. It's obsessional, exhausting, it strains every relationship you have, it's odd, you don't fit, it feels mad and weird or hysterically funny, and all the time you are working against your own and everyone else's conditioning, which says you shouldn't be doing this thing that matters so much. In the midst of all my waiting, of course, heterosexual friends around became pregnant, gave birth, and I couldn't express to them the real extent of my jealousy and fury.*

*My worst time was always the point at which the first period pain told me, so soon, that the hoping was over again this month, and then having to wait for the bleeding, knowing it would come. Every month I felt that I had lost another baby, another one had died. Every month my partner, not quite comprehending my needs but seeing my pain, would hold me until I could face it again. I couldn't let it go, not allowing the possibility that it wouldn't work eventually.*

*In the end we persuaded the donor, already the father of three, to have a sperm count. It turned out to be zilch, so low as to be non-existent. We waited while he got treatment and started again. His wife conceived. I didn't.*

*There were tests and more donors. There was nothing wrong with my body that anyone could tell, but after the laparoscopy\* I'd had enough. After a break of several months, I couldn't face a return to more tears and heartache, and I had a life to live that was now gradually being wasted. I expected sadness and regrets, uncertainty and ambivalence, but that wasn't how it was. After a shaky time and some numbness and distance from it all, I feel as if my hangover is well and truly over. I am well, happy, full of beans, creative and am*

---

\* A *laparoscopy* is an operation where a thin tube is inserted into the abdomen to look at the internal organs, especially the ovaries and Fallopian tubes. A *D and C* is a dilatation and curettage – an operation done under general anaesthetic in which the lining of the uterus is scraped and examined. An *HSG* is a hysterosalpingogram – an X-ray of the Fallopian tubes and uterus done after injecting dye into the uterus and tubes. This is a test to diagnose blocked Fallopian tubes.

*even – amazing thought! – enjoying the glimmerings of relief and pleasure at making plans which don't involve the patter of anybody's tiny feet!*

● *Bev (1992)*

*I have been trying to get pregnant for five and a half years. At first this was through donor insemination at the Pregnancy Advisory Service [PAS]. After eighteen months, I had a progesterone test, which showed that my own progesterone was not high enough to sustain a pregnancy, so I started on Clomid [a 'fertility' drug which induces ovulation] on days 2 to 6 of my cycle. I had also been looking for my own donors through advertising, but without success, when a colleague told me of a donor. That seemed OK and she agreed to act as an intermediary for me. I still went to PAS, but this was getting to be unsatisfactory. It was now very expensive, and they told me that the likelihood of conceiving using frozen sperm was only 40 to 60 per cent.*

*For a while I continued only with my 'fresh' donor. Self-insemination was sometimes very frustrating. My cycles are very long and irregular and it was hard to predict when I would be fertile. Being on the Clomid, I was getting better at predicting my ovulation time, but my donor liked to know about a week in advance when he was needed. Adding to this holiday times, illness and when he was away for a weekend, there were many times when I didn't have any inseminations or they were at completely the wrong time.*

*After three years of trying, I asked my doctor to refer me for infertility checks, and I was given an appointment at the hospital. I duly went along, but when the doctor found out I was single, he refused to see me, saying it was the policy of the health authority not to treat single women without partners. A friend of mine who was also suffering infertility problems was under the consultant Wendy Savage and suggested I contact her. Her secretary told me she wouldn't see anyone who lived outside Tower Hamlets, but suggested that I write a letter explaining my situation, backed up by a covering letter from my doctor.*

*In August 1990, I saw Mrs Savage and seven months later I went into hospital for a laparoscopy and D and C, and a month later for an HSG. \* All were normal. Wendy Savage discharged me, telling me to try inseminations for six months and then to try a hostile* *mucus test. Nine months after that, I went for a consultation at another hospital and am now having periodic ultrasound scans to determine the way my cycle works.*

*For the last six months, I have been trying both self-insemination and the 'old-fashioned' method. I met somebody who was willing to be a donor. Rather light-heartedly I told him to start collecting jars (to hold the semen). As it turned out, we didn't need the jars! Now each month I arrange inseminations with my donor of the last three years, as well as 'inseminations' with my donor-cum-lover. He's very eager for me to have a child and wants to be involved with the child in a sort of 'uncle' relationship. I'd like him around more, but it's not possible because he's married. I wouldn't have considered this kind of relationship if it wasn't for the fact that it might be a way to get pregnant. It's also really nice to be sexual again after all these years.*

*The worst thing about trying and waiting for so long is the great feeling of unfairness. I have found my friendship patterns changing as my women friends have started families and have entered a world I am not privy to. I have found it extremely difficult to be with people who have children, and it has seemed like I am the only person who doesn't have a child who wants one, as each of my friends has become pregnant. This has been very painful, but the worst of these was the pregnancy and now motherhood of my best friend. It seemed to change everything. I know she wanted to share her joy with me at being pregnant. She even wanted me to be her birth partner. But she knew that it would hurt me to see her with the thing I had wanted for so long, long before she had even thought of it for herself. This put a strain on our relationship, and as she got to the stage where her pregnancy was beginning to show, I decided not to see her. I thought this would become easier when the child was born, but it hasn't. So she also has crossed the magical divide where I can't follow at the present time. I have not yet come to terms with this and still don't see her.*

*This trying for so long takes a great toll on one's self-confidence. Each month as I bleed, it is a slap in the face to my fulfilment as a woman. It is hard to believe that I can ever get pregnant, and the two-week wait has turned from a time of hope and expectation to one of counting the days until I bleed, so I can start planning for next month.*

*Although my friends are very supportive, not having a partner to share all the intricacies has been noticeable. I feel my* friends don't always want to hear about the little things happening to my body each month that I am only too well aware of. To know that someone is rooting for me as much as I am rooting for myself would be a great asset.

Each month is a grieving for a child who after all this time has almost become real. If I believe in it, it will happen, so each month when I call my child into my body, it is like a death when the blood comes. To give up before my body dictates that I have to is not a consideration for me. If I never have a child I can at least say I tried everything in my power for as long as I could. There is a societal pressure, not least from my mother, that says as I reach 40, I should accept that I'm not meant to be a mother. However, this serves only to make me more determined.

# Chapter eight

# Telling Others

## Telling family

THE announcement of a pregnancy, especially a planned one, is traditionally a cause for celebration. We expect our families to congratulate us and we want them to accept our news without reservation. Most lesbians and single women fear that this won't happen. We can't take for granted the reactions of our parents and other family members. We have to prepare ourselves for breaking the news. We can't automatically look forward to the day with pleasure in case they respond with disapproval and shock. Some women feel anxious, some resentful, some try not to think about it. Everyone develops her own strategy for telling the family, based on what she feels she can cope with and what she anticipates from them.

One approach some women try is to announce their intentions before trying to get pregnant, giving the family plenty of time to come to terms with the idea. This lessens the shock value of presenting them with the accomplished deed, but also gives them time to harden their attitudes against the idea and to put pressure on you to abandon your plans.

Another approach is to announce the news when your pregnancy is confirmed or when you feel you are past the danger of miscarrying. Many women keep very quiet about their attempts to get pregnant, to protect themselves during a potentially difficult time. The thought of dealing with anxious and hostile relatives at this time can be too much to take on. It may also be difficult to cope with during early pregnancy if you are struggling with nausea, exhaustion and feelings of vulnerability.

The reactions may not be as bad as you feared. There are

parents who are delighted to have a grandchild and who aren't concerned that their daughter isn't married or with a man. Even parents who are less than enthusiastic during the pregnancy can change completely when the baby is born and becomes a reality. It is hard for a grandparent to resist the charms of a newborn grandchild.

It may be that you do have a hard time when you tell your family. Many people have never heard of donor insemination or have heard pieces of misinformation about it. They are even less likely to have heard of self-insemination. They may think that you have done something dangerous or immoral. They may be worried how you will manage, but their concern may come across as condemnation instead of caring. They may be especially anxious about what they will tell their friends and relatives. If they have been keeping quiet about your lesbianism or your unmarried status, they will find it particularly hard to explain a baby. They may feel that your decision has put them in a difficult position and that they will have to defend your choice to their friends. If you choose or feel forced to reveal that you are a lesbian at this stage, you will have to deal with their possible homophobia as well as their reactions to a lesbian being a mother. Not all lesbians do come out to their family or feel that it is necessary, even when they are planning to have a child.

### ● Hazel (1991)

*I came out to my mum before I left Canada six years ago. Then I met Donna over here. By the time they met Donna they knew she was my partner and that we'd be together for a long time.*

*We'd been talking about getting pregnant for a couple of years. About six months before we were going to do it, I'd been checking my cycle. My mum and dad were over to visit. I told them we were going to start trying. It worked so quickly, the first time. I phoned my parents and said it worked. My mum said, 'Oh my God. So fast!'*

*My parents are very supportive. They always have been. My mum was here for the birth. They're both tickled pink.*

### ● Rose (1992)

*I've never really properly come out to my family because I'm still angry with my mother. In my first lesbian relationship, my mother found and read letters of mine and did a whole number on me until I told her it would never happen again. I've got to tell them first of all that I'm a lesbian, because as long as I don't say it, they can pretend I'm not. Then I've got to say that Iona is my lover. I've got to do all that yesterday because next I've got to tell them about Iona getting pregnant and that might happen tomorrow. I feel under pressure.*

*My sister-in-law is pregnant. One day, I was visiting my sister when she was digging children's things out of the loft to give to my sister-in-law. There were toys, clothes and children's furniture, and I thought, 'Wait a minute. I want some of that for our child.' I said, 'Iona's thinking of having a child.' I've never actually told my sister what my relationship with Iona is about, though I think she knows. Because I haven't properly come out, everyone pretends it's not happening. My sister then asked, 'Is she thinking of getting married then?' She was bewildered even though she knows full well that that's not the case. Perhaps she thought that was the right thing to say. When I said no, she asked who the boyfriend was. I said, 'There's no boyfriend and she's not with a man. That's not how she's going to have a child. She's going to artificially inseminate.' My sister just looked at me and finally said she couldn't agree with it. I replied, 'I'm not asking you to agree with it. I'm just telling you. I'm going to be helping Iona bring up our child.' I was thinking to myself, 'I'm not asking you to agree with it. I'm just asking you to give me that cot. It looks really nice,' but I didn't say that. She looked at me as if I had just landed from outer space and said, 'Oh I just can't agree with this at all. A child should have a mother and a father.' I said, 'What does that say about me? Am I freaky Rose? My dad died when my mum was expecting me so I never had a father figure.' She said, 'Oh but your mother never had a choice.' I came back with, 'So we shouldn't have choices?' But that was it. She wouldn't talk about it any more.*

*Since then, neither my sister nor anyone in my family has said anything about it or asked if Iona is pregnant yet. Nevertheless I'm supposed to think it's all wonderful that my sister-in-law is due in April.*

● **Bev: Conversation with mother (1986)**

Bev: 'I didn't want to tell you before because I didn't know how you'd react, but I'm going to try to have a baby.'

Mother: *(Absolute silence)* 'Well, I am getting on a bit. I've probably only got another ten years to spend with my grandchildren. It's your life. I can't tell you what to do. How are
you going to do it?'

Bev: 'I'm going to a clinic.'

Mother: 'Do you have to pay for it?'

Bev: 'Yes, it's going to cost quite a lot.'

Mother: 'Are you sure you're doing the right thing? Don't you
think you'll ever meet somebody?'

Bev: 'I might do, but I'm getting older and it might be in twenty
years' time.'

Mother: 'But you'd just have to go out with a man for a night!'

Bev: 'I would think that is very hypocritical.'

Mother: 'Why pay out all that money? It's not very natural, is it?'

### (1987, 1988, 1989, 1990, 1991)

Mother: 'What are you doing, still trying to get pregnant? You are
just selfish. All you want is the experience of being pregnant.
You don't care about anyone but yourself.'

Bev: 'Yes, I do want the experience of being pregnant. But that's
only a part of it. I have a much more long-term perspective
than that. I think I know what children are all about. After
all, I work with them. I know what they're like.'

Mother: 'That's different. You don't know anything about it.
Anyway, you're coming up to 40. You're too old to have a
child.'

Bev: 'You were older than 40 when you had me.'

Mother: 'That's different.'

### ● Bronwen (1986)

When I was first pregnant and on holiday alone with my
mother, I didn't tell her, although we were far from home and I was
bursting to tell someone. I waited a few weeks until we had
returned and I was sure of the pregnancy, then phoned her up, with
my best friend sitting holding my hand on the sofa beside me for
support. Self-insemination is less of an issue with her, I think, than
choosing to be a single parent and involve no father. I knew I'd
need support because at that time her comments could have really
got to me. They tapped my own unspoken ambivalences and fears

*about managing alone. So I introduced the topic by saying brightly, 'And now I've got some brilliant news and you're going to be really pleased, or else, so sit down. I'm going to give you your first grandchild.' Apparently my sister phoned her later that day saying, 'Isn't it wonderful news!' and gave her a lecture about not loading her worries and negative feelings on to me, but just to welcome the child.*

● *Sue (1986)*

*When I told my mother, she was fairly upset, though she tried not to show it, which is her way. Even though Benji is a year old now, I don't think that really she has come to terms with it fully, though she treats him the same as my sister's children, and we don't argue about it or anything like that.*

*My father on the whole was much more accepting. He made a joke about his other son-in-law being a test tube, but otherwise he didn't say much to me. But during the time I was pregnant and having the baby, he was dying of cancer, so perhaps that made him much more accepting, more pro-life in general and less concerned with oppressive moral attitudes. He died when Benji was three months old, and he told me how glad he was that he had lived long enough to see him born. His genuine and warm acceptance of Benji is now a big part of my memory of my father.*

● *Shaheen (1992)*

*I've been a lesbian for about twenty years. When I first came out to my mum, she was very supportive. I can remember the words she said to me: 'Well, I can't give you a good example of heterosexual life and marriage. Look at me.' When my parents got divorced, she had a harrowing time emotionally. My parents fought for years. She was going through emotional hell. She's always been tremendously supportive of me. She has been to gay clubs with me when I was younger.*

*My mum knows all the ins and outs of how I got pregnant. She was absolutely fascinated. I think that she was very pleased in a way, seeing that I was taking control myself and was not reliant on a man except for the sperm. All my family know, but they don't all talk about it. No one ever asks where Anton actually came from. My family were very supportive and protective of me when my girlfriend, Jackie, left. My mum was very worried and really felt for me, because she was a single parent when she had my older brother. My sister wanted to ring Jackie up and give her a rocket. I said I didn't think that would be very constructive. They related to it as if it was just like a heterosexual situation where you've been ditched by a man.*

● Toni (1986)

*My plan was to tell my parents when I was already well pregnant. I had been dropping hints for many months beforehand, but the only reaction I got from my mother was, 'Oh, you don't want a child. You're a career woman.' She knew I was a lesbian and it sounded to me like she needed to categorize me as a career woman in order to accept that I wasn't going to have a husband and a family.*

*When I did get pregnant, I felt unsure about it for many weeks because I kept bleeding slightly. I didn't tell my parents. Then I miscarried one day and, by chance, my parents phoned me for a chat that very day. I couldn't say anything while I was feeling so miserable. All I needed was sympathy, but I couldn't be sure that's what I'd get. However, I felt angry not to be able to talk to them about it. I then wrote a very long letter to my mother explaining in great detail why I wanted a baby and how I was going about it. I described the method of self-insemination, leaving nothing to the imagination. She later told me that she was so shocked after she got the letter that she was speechless. (This is actually an unheard of state for my mother.)*

*During the pregnancy, she was extremely negative and worried. She wanted me to have an amniocentesis and was appalled at my plans to have a home birth. Luckily she lives far away and couldn't influence me too much. When Claire was born, she switched over from absolute anxiety to total ecstasy. Since then, I've really appreciated her love for Claire and her acceptance of us.*

● (1991)

*When Claire was 2, we were on holiday together with my parents in Berkeley, California, a place with a large population of self-inseminating lesbians. We went to a public swimming pool where my mother struck up a conversation with a woman carrying a baby. I've never understood how my mother managed to bring it into the conversation but I overheard her saying brightly, 'So how did you get that baby?' The woman replied evasively that she grew it herself. This was probably designed to deter further questions, but she hadn't reckoned on my mother. Without batting an eyelid, my mother said, 'You mean you did self-insemination! I know all about that. My daughter got her baby by self-insemination. See that little girl in the pool. She's the cutest thing that ever lived.'*

● *Paula (1991)*

My mother is as accepting as she can be. The first time I told her about self-insemination, she told me that a child needs a father. I said, 'Is that so? In most heterosexual relationships, children don't have fathers.' She said they would in an ideal world. I said that we don't live in an ideal world. She has the heterosexual fantasy of the family even though she had a totally dismal marriage. It was a big mistake. I was about 9 when my father left us. But she doesn't refer to it now at all. I only see my father occasionally. He hasn't met my daughter, Tara.

My mother is very much into Tara. She usually comes up three or four times a year and spends time with us. She recognizes Nicole's role, though when she's here, she tends to refer to me all the time. I keep saying to her that she can ask Nicole. Nicole's mum is also very supportive and sends Tara Christmas presents. Tara has been up there loads of times.

● *Mike (1991)*

I mentioned to my mother that I was considering being a donor and she was absolutely appalled. She said that gay people and lesbian people do not have children, that the children are going to be brought up to be queers. I asked her where I and all these gay people come from? They must have had straight parents.

She was horrified at the thought of me being a donor, at the thought that she might have grandchildren and not know about them. It's an unmentionable subject now. I wouldn't talk about it with her any more. I'm sad in a way, because I'm usually quite open with my parents. I don't think being a donor is anything to be ashamed of. My parents have different lifestyles and they've been brought up to get married and have children, and if you don't go *along with that, they think you shouldn't have children. They've got used to me being gay. I don't care what they think about that. As far as I'm concerned, I've got my own life to lead. I don't see any reason why parents should hold on to their children. I was brought up to be independent. It's my life.*

## Telling friends and acquaintances

Sooner or later, you will probably be asked by someone who the father of your child is, especially if there's no man around. If you are heterosexual, people will most likely assume that you became pregnant during a relationship with a man which has since broken down. You will have to make a conscious effort to challenge this if you want them to think otherwise. The same is true for single lesbians. Unless there is an obvious woman lover in your life, most people, including other lesbians, wouldn't consider the possibility that you might be a lesbian. The presence of a child usually blocks people from suspecting that you are, and makes it possible for you to pass as heterosexual. This has its disadvantages in that you can end up feeling invisible as a lesbian mother. Lesbians who are open about their sexuality are likely to be asked how their baby was conceived, and have to face the many possible reactions other people have to donor insemination and lesbian motherhood.

There are so many different situations where the issue of telling or not telling comes up that it's not possible to work out a strategy for every one. Sometimes a situation arises and in a split second you have to decide what and how much to tell. There are times when it's easier to let people believe what they want to believe than to launch into the minefield of explaining donor insemination. With friends and workmates, you will probably feel most comfortable once you are clear in your own mind how open you are going to be. There are bound to be surprises, both pleasant and unwelcome ones, even from people you thought you knew well.

● *Sue (1986)*

*I wouldn't say that many of my friends appeared surprised because for years I'd been saying I intended at some point to have a child. Living in London in recent years, it has become the case that more lesbians are having babies in this way. Many of my friends were therefore prepared and pleased for me. I work in a left-wing organization in the voluntary sector, so that isn't really a hostile climate. Even so, because I am an 'out' lesbian at work they were all very startled when I announced my pregnancy. I have found that since Benji was born, I have become more guarded with the infor-mation, because it is his now as well as mine, and as he gets older and begins to understand things, that will be even more the case.*

### ● Pat (1986)

*I don't tell anybody, except for my friends. I've got one old school friend who knows that I'm a lesbian and that I had Marcy through AID. My sister's the only family I have, so I told her. But she knew I was a lesbian anyway. She's married with two children and her husband knows. All my lesbian friends know.*

*But people to do with outside – all the straight people I have to meet – I don't tell them anything. If it comes down to it in conversation, something about fathers, I just say I had a relation-ship with a man and I don't see him any more, which is quite common anyway. It happens all the time. And the clinic, they just think it was a relationship that broke down. So did the hospital. I wouldn't mind telling them, but I couldn't be bothered with the hassle, if there was any, plus being single and on Social Security. I'd rather they just didn't know. It's none of their business. But it is hard, because they always ask about the father when you get preg-nant. I'd rather be able to tell the truth, but it's easier to say the relationship broke down.*

### ● Laura (1992)

*I don't 'tell' others.*

*Although I don't want to be seen as a lesbian who had a child by a father who is no longer around, the child for example of a marriage (and sometimes I do tell people I was married), neither do I think the time is ripe for telling people, outside close friends, about how I conceived Jenny. It is her experience, her creation that is relevant here, and truths she will live with in her own way. I don't feel the need to broadcast to the world about insemination. She has to deal with having a disability and having two lesbian mothers. I don't need to add on that her conception was by donor. It's up to her.*

I had a funny experience in relation to Jenny's primary school, the kind of experience I've never had anywhere else in all the time I've been a lesbian. Maybe I've been lucky or maybe I've avoided trouble. Maybe people swear at me behind my back but I've never had direct experience of abuse, except in the street.

In the first term of my daughter's first year at school, I helped in the classroom one morning a week, every week. They were glad to get the help and I felt it was my contribution to her getting settled at school. The teacher was very traditional, as it turned out. Her teaching seemed very restricted to me. I found the teacher peculiar. She had a twitch in her eye, a sort of nervous tic which meant she couldn't look directly at you. She looked sideways and her eyes fluttered all the time. I felt sorry for her and took no notice.

We were not happy with the school for many reasons, and only carried on because a new headmistress was promised and we felt she might sweep away all the rather bad teaching that went on. At the beginning of the next term, we made an appointment to see the new headmistress, to check her out. She was extremely nice, very approachable, very warm. As usual, three of us, all 'mothers', had come to the meeting, two of us lesbians and one not, so we all crowded into the head's room and she seemed little bothered. Very quickly I made a decision to come out and did so. No problem. I offered to lend her certain books and said I wanted to 'come out' to my daughter's teacher. 'Well', she said, 'I don't know my staff very well yet. Let me suss out the situation and talk to you about it again.' I agreed, for her, not for us, and off we went.

I was surprised the next day by her calling to me at the door of the school. She handed me back the books I'd lent and said, 'Oh, by the way, about the other question ...'

'What other question?' I said, completely puzzled.

'About you being lesbian mothers.'

'Yes?' I said.

'Well, I've spoken to your daughter's teacher' (I felt a bit miffed about that because I'd said I would talk to her), 'and she says that's OK with her, but she's a bit worried about Jenny going round telling all the children that she's a lesbian. She's afraid the other parents won't like it.'

I don't know how this conversation ended. I was stunned.

*First of all, it explained instantly why this teacher was incapable of looking me in the face. She'd known since I first arrived amongst her little reception class that I was a lesbian and it was me she couldn't look at. Yes, she really couldn't look me in the eye. I couldn't believe that anyone could feel so frightened of looking at a lesbian! And of course the other aspect was that my 4¾-year-old really had been going round saying she was a lesbian.*

● *Linda (1986)*

I used to mix with a lot of lesbians in the union. All the lesbian and gay events are very good, because they have very excellent crèches. So in that circle it's quite accepted – certainly in organizational terms. I think in people's heads it's not. If you don't have children, you just have a different pattern of living. And hours mean quite different things. Among gay men I've found there's very little understanding of children. My partner, Margaret, in particular has quite a lot of gay male friends, and I think they're just not into babies or children. I'm a bit disappointed, only in the sense that I would quite like to know more gay men who are perhaps interested in children. It would be nice for Sarah and me.

Having been so long without children, I suppose I'm very used to that way of thinking. It is amazing how if you don't have children, you don't see them. I used to see these little blobs! But I didn't really what I call 'see' them. It's the grossest sort of prejudice! I couldn't tell one baby from another! I was amazed actually that that was the first thing that really struck me when Sarah was born. I couldn't believe it. So I do feel I understand the position of women who haven't got children. And also I do respect women who have chosen not to have children, because there's such a lot of pressure on most women – not on lesbians, but on most women – to have kids. And if you don't have children, I think you have to face quite a lot of hostility from families and society at large. So I always try and remember that, and if they come round, I don't just talk about Sarah. There is a temptation to just talk about the kids and nothing else. So I try and avoid that.

I've told people at work. I try and make myself tell people, because I feel that the more it's discussed, the more acceptable it is, and it becomes part of common experience. And at the end of the day that will make life easier for Sarah. I feel that I'm in a generally privileged position in society. I've got quite a good job and I feel *quite confident. So I don't expect that I'm going to get any shit. I think it is a class thing partly. I think generally middle-class people get better treatment from doctors and various officials.*

*I find it more difficult in just casual encounters. Say I'm with Sarah on the bus, and somebody says, 'I bet you've got your daddy's eyes!' or something like that. Something about daddy. I find that you can't launch into an explanation. I mean, what can you say? Just sort of smile and end it. I find those situations more difficult to deal with.*

● Claire (age 7) 1992

*At school one day we had an assembly about families. My teacher asked me if I would stand up and talk about my family. I didn't mind. I told everyone that I have three mummies and a daddy. I live with my mummy Toni and her girlfriend Theresa, who is my mummy too. I also have a part-time mummy, Marie, who I live with some of the time. Marie has a new girlfriend. My daddy, Pierre, lives with his boyfriend and I like them both a lot. After I told everyone about my family, lots of children raised their hands to ask me questions. One boy asked the first question. He wanted to know how many cars our family has. I was going to count them but my teacher said that the assembly was about families, not about cars. Someone else asked which mummy had sexed with my daddy to make me. I said that they didn't sex, that Pierre put the sperm in a jar. Another boy asked, 'Shouldn't some of those people be married to each other?' I said, 'No, they don't have to. They can do what they want.'*

● Mary (1986)

*I have occasionally talked to heterosexual women about how Owen was conceived. I present it in a very factual way. I think they are terribly intrigued and generally quite shocked, but reluctant to show that because they are all very liberal-minded people. Certainly they are absolutely fascinated by the process. I think that they wouldn't express any hostility towards me, if they felt it. I give them no possibility, no scope to do that. I don't want to hear it. They can work those things out among themselves without me bothering to deal with it. So I just say this is the way it happened. If they're interested, I'll explain more. I'm not into letting them explore their fears around that, their homophobia basically.*

*The only place where fatherhood is an issue is at school. Pete has several times drawn pictures of his 'father' that he's brought home from school. He's also drawn pictures of his 'father' in some terrible accident like a car crash, which is presumably some kind of explanation for why he doesn't have a father. It's an indication of the strength of the pressure coming from school to have a father that he can account for, that he can wipe off if necessary by killing him in a car crash. The pressure is very, very strong. I feel very angry about it. They never talk about fathers or draw them in car crashes when they're among people who know their background. It's only at school they're worried about not having a father. It's like black children drawing pictures of themselves with a white face and hands.*

*Every two or three months, a group of children will come rushing up to me on the playground and say, 'Pete says he's got two mums but he hasn't, has he? It's not true, is it? He hasn't got two mums!' So I just say, 'Yes, he does have two mums. There's me and Barbara who he also lives with.' Then I have a discussion with them about what's a mother and we talk about how a mother might be the person who bore that child, but, for example with children who are adopted, they have a mother who didn't give birth to them but she's still a mother. A mother is somebody who cares for the child and has a responsibility. The children accept that pretty quickly and so, for the next few months, everything is quite calm and dies down.*

*With the teachers, the same kind of things come up. They'll refer to me as Owen's mother, to Barbara as Pete's mother. I keep insisting that I'm Pete's mother too and Owen's other mother is Barbara. They just won't take that on. They refuse to use 'mother' in connection with a non-biological parent. They don't say they won't but they just nod and look a bit embarrassed and change the subject, and carry on doing exactly as they were doing before. There's an enormous amount of resistance from the teachers and absolutely no support at all in terms of getting other children to recognize alternatives to heterosexuality.*

*Ultimately what it means is that Pete and Owen are having to cope with this heterosexism within the school and having to challenge it the whole time. They have to say, 'But I have got two mums, so what of it?' They're not getting one ounce of support from anyone in the school for doing that. I feel very bitter they're having to take on the whole weight of heterosexism from such an early age, from 5 years old. There are no books showing children with lesbian mothers. The teachers aren't standing up in front of the class and saying that in a family you might have a father or you might just have a mother or be looked after by several people and some mothers are lesbians. Everybody just lives in different ways. Primary schools could be doing so much towards supporting children of lesbians. Not only are they not supporting them but they've made it very, very clear that they just think that it's a bit odd and even dangerous.*

### ● Bronwen (1992)

We're very lucky that the school Rhys is at wouldn't dream of making presumptions about children having dads or not having two mums. So he's able to blossom in that atmosphere. It's not an issue in that school. Rhys seems completely impervious to teasing by other kids. He's very confident about the explanation now. Usually it comes up when people ask if David or Donald is his dad. He says, 'No, they're my friends. I haven't got a dad as such. I've got a father who gave the sperm to my mum and he lives in X.' Lately I heard him calling his biological father his 'birth father'.

### ● Mike (1991)

I talk to anyone about being a donor because I think it should be talked about. The longer people hush-hush it, the longer it will take for it to be as acceptable as anything else. It just seems so normal. I don't see why there should be any problem. At first, people's reaction is surprise, but once you explain that the woman is a lesbian and that she doesn't want to sleep with a man, then they're quite understanding about it. I do quite a bit of educating people about it. Most of the people I've talked to about it don't know it exists. Some people thought I was donating to a clinic. Most of my friends are women, apart from a couple of men friends. They all feel fine about it.

### ● Judy (1986)

Most of the people who we work with know that Kath, my lover, and I are bringing up our daughter Ruth together. Some of them know we did SI. I get lots of support at work – including *childcare. I'm lucky. I work in a collective where children are welcomed and there are other lesbians.*

*Some people know more than others. I'm selective about how much I say depending on who I'm talking to. But I don't believe in making up stories about it. I tell the truth – but sometimes only part of it. Why not? Heterosexual women don't go around saying, 'I screwed to get pregnant.' It's assumed. I won't always say I did SI, but I would deny that I had sex with a man or that Ruth has a father. Sometimes I say something like 'I'm bringing her up with the woman I live with' or 'The father is not around' (if they're really persistent). If I feel OK about it, I say I conceived her through SI or AID (as they're more likely to understand that term).*

*I haven't had that much negative feedback on doing SI. I did get criticism from women, especially lesbians, for wanting to get pregnant. They implied I would be wasting time on children. I got hostility in the form of questions like 'What will you do if it's a boy?' from some feminists. I have experienced other people's doubts about SI, bordering on hostility, in the form of questions about the baby wanting/needing a father. It seems like I've lost a lot of lesbian and other friends since having a baby. Maybe because their lives don't have space for children or me as a mother. I know other women find this. On the other hand I've had support from a lot of other people and got closer to other women and children, especially lesbians who have done SI. I think it's really important that we know each other, for ourselves and our children's sakes. I do worry about how my daughter will cope in the future, about how other people will make her feel about being an SI baby and having two lesbian mothers.*

*I made the decision to do SI with my lover, so we both discussed this and felt strongly that our child should be brought up by two mothers with no hint of a 'father'. Already my feelings about this are confirmed. From birth, the comments about the baby have been to do with how much she looks like me (or my lover). Nothing ever enters our heads or is said by people around us regarding whether she looks like someone else – because none of us know. It is a non-issue!*

*People always want to know what I will do about telling our daughter when she is older. I can only trust that I made the right decision, to tell the truth. At one stage I thought I would have to make up stories, but now I realize that's stupid.*

● *Kath (1986)*

*Judy and I are very clear that we're both mother. It's mainly straight friends who have found it easier to accept me as Ruth's mother. They find it easier to accept us if they see us in a heterosexual way which gives me that status. It's double-edged. They definitely see me as mother. The shit that we've had, and there has been some, is mainly from lesbian friends. They're the ones who say things to Ruth like 'Are you going to go to your mum or are you going to go to Kath?' They can't quite take it on. It makes me feel angry rather than anything else. It's an embarrassment too sometimes – feels like I'm being dismissed. I do as much for Ruth. I have as many sleepless nights, I wash as many nappies. I take as much of the responsibility as Judy does. A lot of childless lesbians just don't know what childcare is about. I guess that's why heterosexual mothers find it easier to accept us. A lot of them are jealous. To them, the idea of two women bringing up a child is wonderful. It's totally clear to them.*

● *(1992)*

*When we try to establish if Ruth has any aggro from other children at school about her family, she just says that she has two mummies and tells them to go away. She has never displayed any jealousy of any of her friends who have fathers, or any sense of unease at having two mummies. Fathers just don't seem to be an issue for her at this point in time.*

# Dealing with the medical profession

Compared to donor insemination through clinics, self-insemination is a process which takes the control of fertility away from the medical profession and puts it into women's hands. Because of this and because it is mostly lesbians who are doing self-insemination, many members of that profession are hostile to the idea and to the practice, assuming that they have even heard about it. There are, of course, progressive and supportive GPs, midwives and consultants, some of whom have even been known to recommend donor insemination to their lesbian patients or who have done self-insemination themselves. Without having carried out a large-scale survey, I suspect that they are still a small minority, probably concentrated in big cities. In general, there are still grounds for suspicion about the attitudes of the medical profession.

The best and probably only way of finding out what attitudes medical practitioners have is through word of mouth. You can learn a lot by talking to lesbian mothers and other women who have done self-insemination about their experiences with particular doctors and midwives in your area. It is worth going out of your way to see a sympathetic GP if you can. Practically speaking, this is not always possible. It may be that you don't know any other lesbian mothers who can give advice, or the choice of medical practitioners in your area may be very limited. The best you can do then is to work out a strategy and see what happens. One tactic to consider for the birth is to name your partner or friend on your birth plan as your birth partner. This gives that person a status that should be recognized and respected, especially if you need any emergency medical care.

There is no medical reason why any member of the medical profession should know that your child was conceived by self-insemination. It is as relevant to the clinical care they will be providing as whether or not you had an orgasm at the time of conception. It helps to remember that self-insemination is essentially a private, non-medical act. The knowledge that you are pregnant as a result of self-insemination should not influence the advice they give you. They may act as if it is important for them to know all about what you did. They may claim that it was dangerous to do it on your own, that you could cause damage to yourself or your child through injury, infection or genetics. In the context of the known dangers of sexual intercourse, these claims make no sense. Unfortunately, knowing that you have done self-insemination may influence their attitude towards you and thus the quality of care. You may feel very vulnerable to the medical profession in the course of pregnancy and birth. Having unsympathetic medical staff who disapprove of what you have done is not going to help.

There is always the possibility that the information will end up on your medical records and eventually on your child's. Once it is on your records, you will be powerless to do anything about it, and future doctors may make judgements about you as a result.

● *Hazel (1991)*

For the most part, everyone I had contact with, whether they knew I was lesbian and had done self-insemination or didn't, were positive in every respect that I can imagine. The only exceptions were the doctors at the end of the delivery, who whisked in and whisked out, which I suspect is fairly typical. Before I even got pregnant I was thinking how I would deal with the doctors and the midwives and everyone else involved. I was almost ready to have to fight or to argue, to feel defensive, and I didn't have to do any of that with anyone at all. I was a bit paranoid, thinking all I needed was one panicked midwife in the hospital, who would send the welfare woman around and start deciding Jordan was at risk for some bizarre reason. I was a bit worried about that, but after I was introduced to my midwife, I didn't get that feeling again.

I decided that I would neither stay in the closet nor wear a big 'L' on my forehead. If my lesbianism was an issue, we would talk about it. If it wasn't, then it wouldn't matter. That's why in some cases, the midwives don't know, and it's not on my forms and that's fine. But I thought it was important for the midwives I saw all the time and who I thought might deliver Jordan to know, specifically because of Donna, my partner. If I had been on my own, it might not have mattered quite as much for them to know, but because Donna is such an important part of my life, I wanted them to know. She wasn't just a birth partner. She is my partner. She was there not just in the capacity of wiping my brow while I was having contractions but as part of Jordan's life.

Right from the beginning I put down Donna as my next of kin. The community midwife saw it and asked if I would like to bring her along to the next clinic. She asked whether the father had hereditary illnesses or conditions that she should know about. I said, 'Not to my knowledge.' She said, 'You don't know him very well, do you?' I told her that I had used artificial insemination. She was really interested and didn't get freaked out. I had been a bit nervous of what she might say.

The main midwife made a point of being my midwife right through the whole pregnancy. She set up special appointments for me so that I would only see her. They didn't have to do that. I would have found it a lot harder if I had had to keep explaining my situation to each and every midwife. She and the student midwife tried to make things easy for me and Donna, much easier than I *was expecting. They would talk about Martina [Navratilova] to make me feel comfortable.*

The student midwife who was with her at the time wanted to interview me for her midwifery course, as she was doing a paper on the special needs of minority groups. She was finding that her fellow classmates were not dealing with the minority groups in London very well at all. So she interviewed me and Donna and took it to the rest of the midwives in her class. Apparently it went very well.

The midwives in the hospital were really supportive of Donna. They included her in all the decision-making. I set up a birth plan and requested specifically that Donna be included in the decision-making – that she was to make decisions if I wasn't able to. They respected that. After Jordan was born, my midwife came into the hospital to see me. She hadn't been there for the delivery. The student midwife was there during the delivery for longer than an eight-hour shift. She stayed as an observer and for support. That was nice.

The obstetrician finally came round and asked me what sort of contraception I'd like, and I said I didn't want any. He asked if I was having another baby then. I told him I'm a lesbian and won't need contraception. He said fine. He didn't fall off the bed or put a big scarlet 'L' on my forms. I was quite pleased.

### ● Mary (1986)

During my pregnancy, I didn't explain to my GP or to anyone how Owen had been conceived. I simply said I didn't know who the father is. He's not around and that's an end to it. My lover at the time was included in the visits, and the GP knew that she was my lover, although we didn't talk openly about being lesbians. The doctor was pretty good about it. He didn't push me to explain.

However, after Owen was born and it became apparent that he was different from other children, I started going to specialists. The first visit I made to a consultant was a complete shock. I thought that the only information he had about me was the letter that I was carrying from my GP, and which I knew just said something like 'Mother is worried about this child. Please investigate.' But after the specialist had spoken to me for a while, it was obvious there was something he wanted to say but was finding difficult to get out. He finally said that he'd heard Owen might have been conceived by AID. I was completely thrown. I managed to say that I didn't want to comment on that.

But on the next visit, having thought about it, I felt, well, if he knows, I'd rather he also knows that I feel fine about self-insemination and that it wasn't a problem for me. I didn't want to be put on the defensive. So I said, 'Yes, in fact he was conceived by self-insemination, but I want to know how you got that information. Was it from my GP?' He wouldn't tell me but he insisted it wasn't my GP. I went on assuming it was, until it transpired that it was a health visitor who I'd had some contact with about a community project that we were both involved in.

The doctor wanted to know all sorts of details, like how many men I had had sperm from at the same time – things that were completely irrelevant to what had happened to my child (he'd been affected by a Cytomegalovirus infection during the pregnancy). It's partly that he didn't know what to ask, partly voyeurism. But it was all expressed with an absolutely straight face on his part. Each question was put as if it were as valid as the next and as if he knew exactly why he was asking it. It was as if he had an absolute right to ask anything he wanted. I refused to give any information about the donors. He didn't pronounce any moral judgements on what I'd done, but behind his facade of professionalism was an awful lot of antagonism. It was obvious he was going to go away and discuss it with as many people as he thought appropriate, and the words 'lesbian' and 'AID' would be written prominently in the file. I knew that and I've had to accept the consequences.

For a long time after, I felt incredibly insecure. The consequences for me were that I felt pressure to be as 'normal' as possible and to prove that I was a 'good mother'. For a couple of years after Owen was born, I felt anxious whenever I had to go to doctors. When I took Owen for hospital appointments I wore a skirt instead of trousers, which I wear the rest of the time. I just had one skirt. I couldn't bring myself to iron it or to wear nylon tights, so I always looked a bit odd. I couldn't say anything foolish in front of them. I really had to be on top of what I was doing.

I was constantly worried that someone might decide we weren't really fit to be Owen's mothers. This was especially true because I had very different views from the doctors about disability – like insisting Owen had the right to stay in the community and not to be forced into segregated nurseries or schools. The doctors *thought my views were naive or irresponsible (though of course they never said this openly). They also thought I was ready to 'sacrifice' Owen for the sake of my political principles. The combination of that and our being lesbians left me feeling very unsafe, even though I always believed that they wouldn't win. It had a very profound effect on me, and my lover used to tell me that I behaved in a peculiar way before I went to see doctors. It was because of that anxiety. Now I feel a lot more confident about my ability to carry it off, as it were, as a lesbian who has a child with disabilities.*

● *Linda (1986)*

*I did tell the hospital and my doctor in the clinic. I was at a terribly trendy, 'right-on' health centre. They said, 'Oh yes! Wonderful! How interesting! You should have done it on the National Health.' But I didn't consider it because I didn't imagine it to be possible.*

● *Pat (1986)*

*I don't think I'm on the same level at all with my doctor, so it's hard for me to admit certain things. Because why did I have an AID baby? It's because I'm a lesbian. And they don't think I'm a lesbian. I don't want them to know because of my children, really. It probably would have been all right for me to say it, as I like my doctor a lot, but I don't feel that I could just say it. I'm always so scared that something could happen. But you do have to come out with all silly stories instead!*

● *Judy (1986)*

*In the hospital I said I didn't know who the father was. My lover came to most of the appointments and was noted in my records as co-parent. The (male) consultant realized we were lesbians but didn't let on until the last appointment, when the baby was just overdue. He asked a medical student present how one could help bring on labour. The (male) medical student said, 'Sex, because of the prostaglandins in the semen.' The consultant asked him, 'What if the mother is gay?' The student was speechless. The consultant replied that female orgasm could also help produce prostaglandins and induce labour.*

*I was booked for a GP delivery, and the doctors knew I'm lesbian and that was OK. The midwives were very nice and the question never arose, although it was obvious on home visits that there wasn't a father around. The health visitors know that I'm bringing my child up with a woman and I think they know I'm a lesbian, but it doesn't seem to affect how they treat me. As far as the medical profession is concerned I've not had any problems.*

*Generally I'm careful because I don't want to encourage homophobia. I'd rather people accepted me and then found out I was a lesbian. At the same time I'd never pretend that there is a father involved, and I always am honest about living with a woman who is also our child's mother, and that I did SI.*

● *Sue (1986)*

*I had been in labour for about sixteen hours when I was transferred from home to hospital because the labour was going on too long. When I got to the labour ward, the registrar was taking down my personal details; name, address, occupation, etc. She saw that I had women friends with me and said, 'So there's no man around then?' and I said no. She then said, 'So it's an AID baby then?' I said yes, which I know I shouldn't have done, but I had been in labour for hours, really in pain. I would have said anything at this stage. When my friends later argued with her, she tried to justify it by saying that there are disreputable clinics around and they had to be careful and so on. She also claimed that it was on my GP records, which was untrue. I checked with my GP. When challenged on this, the hospital claimed it was on the community midwives' records, which was also untrue. I hadn't told them either! Some weeks later, I tried to get it removed from the hospital records, but they wouldn't agree, even though my GP was very supportive and wrote to them on my behalf. I feel very angry that I was treated in this way, and furious that they lied to me.*

● *Alex (1991)*

*Because I got sick in the middle of agreeing to be a donor, I was very direct with my doctors. I told them that I was donating sperm to a woman who wants to get pregnant. All of the doctors except one woman were so oppressive. Initially my GP shrugged off the idea of a gay man being a donor. This was when I went to him and he diagnosed me as having hepatitis. He said, 'Have you ever had an HIV test?' I said, 'Yes, yesterday.' He said, 'I wouldn't do it. I wouldn't do it.' He was saying that people like me shouldn't be donors. He wanted to know what hospital I was donating the sperm to. I said no hospital.*

*When I went to a hospital for my hepatitis, the doctor was more or the less the same. First he asked me if I was a passive or an active homosexual. I knew that I couldn't donate sperm at the time (because of having hepatitis) but I wanted to know when it would be safe to do it. They said very little, just dismissed it and asked what hospital I was donating at. I told them I was doing it privately. The doctor just didn't want to help. The woman doctor was very nice. She didn't flinch when I told her and just said I would have to wait for the result showing that I was not a carrier, and after that, it's fine.*

Chapter nine

# Donor Insemination through Clinics

## Advantages

NOT all women feel that self-insemination is their first choice. Many woman would prefer to go to a donor insemination clinic. The advantages are that clinics will be able to do a more thorough job of screening the donors for sexually transmitted diseases, particularly HIV infection, and for certain genetic conditions than most women will. Anonymity is guaranteed and the clinics have reserves of donor sperm, thus eliminating the need to search for donors. By going to an impersonal agency, you are not in the awkward position of asking someone repeatedly for a favour. A semen analysis will be carried out, which will increase your confidence in the donor's fertility (though it doesn't guarantee that he is fertile).

## Disadvantages

While going to a clinic has major advantages over self-insemination, it also has disadvantages.

The service costs a lot of money, especially if it takes more than a few months to get pregnant. At the Pregnancy Advisory Service, which is a non-profit-making charitable trust, the initial consultation costs £165, after which you pay £137 per cycle (prices correct as of December 1993). There were 96 centres throughout the UK licensed to provide donor insemination as of July 1993.

Most of these clinics are private, and some of the NHS clinics charge fees that are nearly as steep as those at private clinics.

Another important disadvantage is that frozen sperm is not as effective as fresh, so that it may take much longer to get pregnant. Moreover, women who want the donor to be involved with the child or to know who he is are out of luck at a clinic. Donors are anonymous and at present no information about him may be given to the children. In the future, Parliament may decide that when children reach the age of 18, they can get hold of certain information about the donor such as eye colour, hair colour, occupation and interests. This information plus the donor's name and date of birth is kept in a central registry by the Human Fertilisation and Embryology Authority. When they reach the age of 16, children can ask whether they or the person they plan to marry was born as a result of donor insemination in a licensed clinic. They will be given a yes or no answer. Even if the law (see next section) is changed in the future to allow clinics to disclose the identity of donors, it will not be retroactive. Anyone donating now will never be identified, though non-identifying information may become available.

The main disadvantage of donor insemination from a clinic is that all decisions about access to 'treatment' are in the hands of the clinic. You are defined as a patient in need of medical treatment, even though your reason for using donor insemination is private and personal and not medical. It has not been easy to find clinics which will provide a donor insemination service to women without male partners. There has been considerable prejudice against lesbians and single women becoming mothers for many years. The Human Fertilization and Embryology Act 1990 has not improved the situation, though it has not made it worse, as was originally feared when the bill was debated in Parliament.

# The Human Fertilization and Embryology Act 1990 (HFEA)

The HFEA brought donor insemination under the control of the state by appointing an Authority (see Appendix A) to grant licences to DI clinics. It is an offence for a clinic to provide a DI service without such a licence. By not complying with the Authority's Code of Practice, a clinic risks losing its licence. Licensing is a way of ensuring that clinics provide an adequate service and are not exploiting their customers.

The Authority does not tell clinics whom to treat or not to treat. There is no statement in either the Act or the Authority's guidelines which says that lesbians or single women cannot receive donor insemination. The doctor in charge of each clinic has the responsibility for deciding who to treat. According to the Authority's guidelines, clinics should not adopt any policy or criterion which appears arbitrary or discriminatory. On the other hand, the Act states that, 'A woman shall not be provided with treatment services unless account has been taken of the welfare of any child who may be born as a result of the treatment including the need of that child for a father.'

This curious, ambiguous statement is a compromise reached after much debate in Parliament. As the bill was going through, there were a number of attempts to ban lesbians and single women from receiving donor insemination services (and the other assisted-conception technologies, such as in vitro fertilization). A House of Lords amendment would have made it an offence for a clinic to provide services to an unmarried couple. This was narrowly defeated, by 61 votes to 60. But at the end of the day, there is nothing in the Act which restricts clinics to heterosexual couples. The Authority's guidelines to clinics are carefully worded to avoid discrimination against lesbians and single women and to make it possible for clinics to provide treatment to them. The guidelines say that in cases where the child will have no legal father,

> centres are required to have regard to the child's need for a father and should pay particular attention to the prospective mother's ability to meet the child's needs throughout his or her childhood, and where appropriate whether there is anyone else within the prospective mother's family and social circle who is willing and able to share the responsibility for meeting those needs and for bringing up, maintaining and caring for the child.

Clinics can interpret this how they like, and will be licensed as long as they can justify their reasons to the Authority. A clinic can say that the lesbian partner is the person in the prospective mother's social circle who will be sharing the responsibility for bringing up the child. The guidelines do not say that this person has to be a man. There are clinics which have taken this position and have been licensed by the Authority. One such is the Pregnancy Advisory Service (PAS – see Appendix A), a non-profit-making charitable trust in London which has been given a licence to provide DI. Its clients include lesbians and single women and the directors publicly said that they refuse to operate a discriminatory service. They satisfy themselves in the initial counselling session that the woman is able to meet the child's needs. They argue that studies suggest that children do not develop abnormally when brought up by lesbians or in single-parent households, so that if a woman can demonstrate that she has thought about the issues and is likely to be an adequate mother, then the clinic has taken into account the child's need for a father.

There was another charitable trust, the BPAS, which openly provided DI to lesbians and single women at eight of its centres in England, Scotland and Wales. Unfortunately it stopped its DI service in July 1991, claiming that it was not cost-effective. This decision coincided with HFEA and with hysterical media coverage about 'virgin births', in which BPAS received much unfavourable publicity. Hopefully it can be persuaded to resume its donor insemination service in the future.

There are also clinics which interpret these guidelines in a homophobic way and use them as a basis for refusing treatment to lesbians and single women. In a meeting with the Authority, I was told that their policy was to encourage clinics not to discriminate against any particular group of women such as lesbians, but that they do not see it as their role to encourage clinics to take a more positive attitude towards treating lesbians and single women. They hope that more lesbians will go to clinics to avoid the risk of HIV through self-insemination. Basically they feel that it is up to each clinic how they interpret the Act and not up to the Authority to tell them who to treat or to steer them in any direction.

It does not appear that the Act has made it any more difficult for lesbians and single women to get donor insemination from a clinic. There are clinics which are doing it, and the situation may even change for the better with enough public pressure from lesbians. It would be better if the Authority took a more positive role in encouraging clinics to adopt less discriminatory policies, but perhaps they too can be persuaded to change.

### Home inseminations

The Licensing Authority is open to the idea of home insemi-nations. This is when a clinic sends the semen to a woman to inseminate herself at home. The woman would still have to be registered for treatment at a clinic and to have passed the initial assessment procedure. She could not be given the sperm still frozen, as that is illegal under the Act, but she could be given it while it was thawing. This would be an advantage for women who do not live near a clinic or who find it hard to get to a clinic because of disability.

### Finding a clinic

The Authority has a list of clinics licensed for donor insemi-nation, but they only give out names and addresses. Even though they have the information on each clinic's criteria for treating women, they do not have it in an accessible form for giving out. Women's Health (see Appendix A) has the same list and tries to keep up to date with each clinic's policies on lesbians and single women. An individual woman can call her nearest clinic and ask for herself what criteria they use. They may reply with the vague remark that they treat each case on its merits or they may be very direct about their criteria.

# Donor insemination in other countries

Compared with other western European countries, Britain is one of the most liberal. In Spain, it is possible for single women to have donor insemination at a clinic but it is not clear whether women who are out as lesbians would. Some countries have no national policies or laws that explicitly deny donor insemination services to lesbians and single women. In Belgium, the Netherlands, Luxembourg and Greece, it depends on the individual clinic, and there are some with enlightened practices. However, in France, Germany, Norway, Portugal, Sweden and Switzerland, lesbians and single women are not allowed access to donor-insemination clinics. There is no common European policy at the moment.

In the USA, there are thousands of doctors and clinics who say they are willing to offer a donor-insemination service to lesbians and single women. There are even more who are opposed, but with a little effort, it is possible to find a supportive service (see the resources section in April Martin's *The Lesbian and Gay Parenting Handbook* for organizations which can help). These services are not cheap and may not be local. Women may have to travel to another state or have frozen semen sent to them through the post. Still, there are many more opportunities for lesbians and single women to organize donor insemination from a sperm bank in the USA than in Britain. One such service is the Sperm Bank of California in Oakland, California, which advertises its donor-insemination programme as being 'for all women, regardless of race, marital status or sexual preference. Women with infertile partners, single women and Lesbians participate'. This sperm bank ships frozen semen specimens in dry ice anywhere in the world to women enrolled in their programme or to medical professionals registered with the sperm bank. The Sperm Bank of California is one of the few clinics in the USA which offers donors the option of either remaining anonymous or of being identified to the children conceived with their sperm when they reach the age of 18. Women choose from a catalogue listing the donors' features and whether they agree to have their identity released.

Many US states have laws which distinguish between sperm donors and fathers. As a donor, a man has no parental rights and responsibilities. To qualify as a donor, most state laws require that the donor insemination be performed as a medical procedure by a licensed doctor on the doctor's premises.

● *Jill (1986)*

*My experiences with BPAS began with the counselling and medical examination which they insist upon and which, in 1983, cost £50. Neither of these was particularly pleasant. The doctor who did the examination was brusque and hardly spoke to me. I had been quite honest about being a lesbian and my lover and I were 'counselled' together. The counsellor, who was quite friendly, asked us why we wanted a child, told us about the procedure of artificial insemination and talked about the implications of having an AID baby. I was frank about the fact that I would prefer a girl, although I was prepared to have a boy. She was obviously con-*

*cerned about this, despite my explanation that I'd thought about it very carefully and over a long period. We talked about our different views of men – a fairly pointless exercise really. I felt the counselling was pretty useless considering that I'd thought about it all at great length, and it certainly didn't bring up anything new.*

*After this, I didn't hear from them for a while, and I started to get suspicious that they hadn't liked my views on the sex of the baby. This was confirmed when I rang them to let them know the results of the rubella immunity test, and a woman grilled me about my opinions of the baby's sex. I simply repeated what I'd said previously, although I felt pretty annoyed about it.*

*They eventually wrote and told me I could start the inseminations the following month, and I did so. The nurse who did the inseminations was fairly friendly, although she rarely volunteered information and I had to ask everything. I would have preferred it had she been more forthcoming.*

*One day she left my lover and me alone with my notes and we read these with great interest. My suspicions that they had thought of turning me down were confirmed, and I felt that they'd twisted round what I'd said about preferring a girl. They said, in the notes, that they were worried that a boy would be rejected! I was really angry, as I'd given no indication of that at all in what I'd said and it was pure speculation on their part. I felt their whole attitude was very anti-lesbian. I didn't see how they could begin to vet the women who came to them for AID, considering that there are so many crucial factors involved in having a child and that any kind of woman can usually get pregnant by intercourse if she chooses. A woman's husband might be a child abuser or they might live in terrible squalor, and how would they check these things out? I feel that if they're offering this type of service, then they have to accept everyone who comes along and who can pay, because any type of screening is completely impractical. I'm pretty sure, had I been in a heterosexual couple, they wouldn't have turned a hair about my preference for a girl.*

*It took me five months to become pregnant and I was getting fairly anxious towards the end because of the cost – £30 per month in 1984. Clinically they're quite thorough, although, as I said, they're not very informative. On the emotional side, they leave a lot to be desired. When I finally conceived, I'd used a donor that a friend had found as well as going to BPAS, and I wondered if conception had finally occurred because I'd used fresh rather than frozen sperm. BPAS say this makes no difference, but I'm not convinced.*

*For the record, I have a beautiful year-old son and we are very happy.*

## ● Pat (1986)

I got pregnant with my daughter Marcy through BPAS. I wouldn't mind a father being involved with Marcy, if only because my older son Dean has got a father somewhere. But I wouldn't want to have a relationship with him to get her. I'd prefer to have no men involved at all. But I would rather have known who Marcy's father was. All I know about him is that he was supposed to be a dark West Indian and that he was probably a medical student.

After being turned down by a black gay men's group, I thought of other ways to find black donors. A friend of mine said that she knew a lesbian who worked for BPAS, and maybe she could ask her. I had thought that only heterosexual women could go there. I didn't think that lesbians could go. She got me an interview. They said it would have to go through a 'board' with a couple of doctors on it to see if they'd accept me.

The first interview was quite OK. They just asked what I wanted and how they could help me, if at all, and why I had come to them. I said that I chose a clinic because I wanted a black donor. However, there were hardly any at the clinic and there were women in line for them anyway. They said there were three women and three donors, plus me.

After that, it got quite difficult, because I had to take the woman I had been having a relationship with for a few years to the interview. I had to force her to go at the time. It took her ages to say that she'd go with me. She went because she knew how much I wanted the baby. I said to her, 'Don't you dare get anything wrong!' She said, 'I won't. I won't.' It was terrible once we were there because we were both trying to say the same thing. Halfway through the interview, they sent me outside and kept my lover there. Then they asked her, 'Do you really want this baby?' And she had to sit there and say, 'Yes, we've thought about it for years now, and we've decided we really, really want to have a baby.' And then she had to go out and I came back in and they asked me the same question.

*We had to be like a husband and wife, and have a home together. They asked me how many 'straight' friends I had, to balance it out I think, and how many men friends I had. We told a lot of lies! We didn't like that at all. But we felt we had to do that to get what we wanted in the end. We were together a few years and were open about being lesbians, so maybe they wouldn't have failed me. It was my last hope, especially wanting a black donor, so I thought if I have to lie my way through, I will. Actually, they were really, really nice, especially my counsellor. They don't discriminate against lesbians at all.*

*After that interview was over, it was very easy. They wrote to me saying they had accepted me. Then I had to go and be examined by the doctor. During all this time I was doing a temperature chart, so I knew when I was ovulating. I would just ring up in the morning when I needed to go up. They said they'd do it for me, but there was a year's waiting list to do it for me at the clinic. So I would take the sperm home in a specimen jar.*

*I used to laugh! I would get on the train with this jar in my pocket and think, 'Oh, my God! If only they knew.' I didn't know whether to rush home or to just go home slowly because it had to defrost. Anyway, I used to rush! I would get home sweating and jump into bed, put it in and then lie there for about half an hour, read a book or something.*

*It's a lot of money. You have to answer questions you know aren't their business and you have to be a file, a case. But they're really friendly and nice and it's good that they don't discriminate against lesbians. Because it's an organization, you can understand them and you tend to trust in them. I did totally. I just assumed that it was totally tested and that it was strong semen and that it was probably the best. It wasn't just somebody I knew as a friend or I didn't know anything about at all.*

*I wrote to them about having a third child. I think it's because I don't have a family, it's just me and my sister. Now I've got a boy and a girl and they say once you've got one of each, you don't want any more. But I do! My counsellor at BPAS is fine about it.*

● *Sharon (1986)*

*First appointment at BPAS for counselling. I spend an hour and a half answering questions about my motives, my emotions, what support I will have, as she tries to find out whether I can cope. Before I went in, I had sat thinking I would have to answer things right, so that they were sure to take me on. I didn't know exactly what the right things to say were, but I knew I would have to find them, much like women needing an abortion and wanting to say the right things to the doctor. But she was so nice, and I answered her truthfully through the whole thing.*

*There were a lot of questions — my family's reactions, my work, whether I would tell anyone what I was doing or keep it a secret. The only question I couldn't answer at all, which I still can't answer, is whether if I got pregnant I would have an amniocentesis and, if it was positive, would have an abortion. It was one of the last questions she asked, and it was a painful one. She also asked if I would want the same man's semen a second time, to have a second child. I said it was all I could do to think about one at this point.*

*She asked if I was sure I didn't want a Jewish donor, and I still feel bad that they didn't have one. She wrote down my characteristics — dark brown eyes and hair, thin, tallish, sallow skin — we had an argument about that. I liked to think of myself as tanned. Sallow sounded so colourless. She said, 'What shall we look for instead of someone Jewish?' and I said, off the top of my head, 'How about Mediterranean?' She said that that shouldn't be too hard and that was that. Later, I asked one of the others there if they kept pictures of the men, not to show the woman, but for their own purposes to match them with the women. They said no. I wanted someone nice looking. I felt guilty for this, as what does it matter, yet when the man is so anonymous as it is, it felt it was the least I could want.*

*We arranged for me to go in a week later, just when my ovulation would have started, so they could do the physical, take a mucus sample and mix it with the semen they had chosen to see if the sperm could swim in it, and to take a blood sample for various tests. They said quite plainly that I would not be able to start on that ovulation and I was royally disappointed. I got over it.*

*The first insemination: the doctor gets me undressed and up on the bed. She puts in the speculum and lets me have a look at my cervix. The first time in my life. I had never got in on any self-examination groups and we have a giggle about that. She takes some mucus. It's clear as a bell. I'm mentally dancing about with the excitement. Then she says, 'Is the speculum hurting? I'll be gone for a few minutes.' When she returns she has a little bottle. I can't see what she is doing over the blanket and I am almost ready to jump about on the table. Then she says quietly that she is putting the semen in with a long, thin catheter, and before I can blink, it is finished and she's taking the speculum out. She tells me to lie there for twenty minutes and she'll be back.*

*It seems so simple. The whole thing feels holy to me, mystical, unbelievable. I am excited, thrilled. I put a pillow under my bum to keep it up there. I had thought she said she had inserted it right into my uterus with the catheter, but later I am told she hadn't. In any case, I didn't leak for the twenty minutes and I lay there wishing the sperm a good journey and willing one of them to connect. I was over the moon.*

*When she came back she brought a rocket cap (to use at home for the next insemination). What a name! She showed me how to use it. Not a word went into my brain. I got dressed and went to work. On the way, the most amazing shudder went through my body. Well, not a shudder exactly, an indescribable feeling of electricity. I thought to myself, 'That was it. It's happened.' But I kept it to myself, as I knew anyone else would say it was absurd.*

*Second insemination (done at home): I go down on the tube to collect the sperm. They tell me to wear a bra because it should be kept warm and it was best either in a bra or in my knickers. Well, not in my knickers, not in the tube. So I put a bra on, which feels awful, and I make sure I pay before they bring it out.*

*When she came out with the little bottle, I grabbed it, shoved it into my bra under my right breast, wondering absurdly whether I should put it on my left side nearer my heartbeat, laughing, and race down the stairs, run to the tube and urge the trains on every second. I keep my right arm tight up against the bottle so it is even warmer and so it doesn't fall out right there in front of the dozy commuters. I race to my house at the other end, sweating and nervous. I get out my syringe, put the rocket cap in, release the sperm into the cap and lie there. I try not to pay too much attention to what I am doing. But the excitement is still there, and after twenty minutes I take it out and a great load of semen and mucus comes with it.*

## Appendix A

# Resources and Reading List

FOR more information on self-insemination groups, donor insemination, pregnancy, infertility, fertility awareness and other women's health issues, contact:

Women's Health
52 Featherstone St
London EC1Y 8RT
Tel. 071–251 6580

## Lesbian parenting

*Considering Parenthood*, by Cheri Pies, 2nd edn, updated. Spinsters Book Company: San Francisco, 1988.

> A very valuable guide for lesbians, giving ideas of exercises to be done in groups or alone which help women clarify their thoughts on a range of issues – being a non-biological mother, adoption, alternative fertilization, co-parenting, single parenting, legal issues, building support networks, choosing not to parent, and more.

*Different Mothers – Sons and Daughters of Lesbians Talk about Their Lives*, edited by Louise Rafkin. Cleis Press: Pittsburgh, 1990.

> These are the accounts of thirty-eight people, ranging in age from 5 to 40, who have grown up in lesbian families. They come from a wide range of backgrounds and talk about what it has meant to them to grow up with a lesbian mother.

*The Lesbian and Gay Parenting Handbook*, by April Martin. Pandora Press: London, 1994.

> The American experience of how lesbians and gay men get children. It covers donor insemination, self-insemination, adoption, surrogacy and co-parenting arrangements with gay men.

*Lesbian Couples*, by D. Merilee Clunis and G. Dorsey Green. Seal Press: Seattle, 1988.

> This book raises many of the issues that lesbians face, such as having children, stages of relationships, living arrangements, work, money and time, resolving conflict, how racism affects couples, and growing older together. It is a sound self-help book with a good bibliography.

*Lesbian Sex*, by JoAnn Loulan. Spinsters Inc: San Francisco, 1984.
This is a practical book for lesbians about lesbian sex, written with the intention of helping lesbians achieve the kind of sex life they want. The chapter on 'Sex and Motherhood' is particularly good but the rest of the book shouldn't be missed either.

*Lesbians Who Are Mothers – Resource List*. Lesbian Information Service, PO Box 8, Todmorden, Lancashire, OL14 5TZ. Tel. 0706–817235. Send £2.
Annotated list of journal articles, chapters in books and books of research about lesbian mothers. Most are from the USA.

*Politics of the Heart: A Lesbian Parenting Anthology*, edited by Sandra Pollack and Jeanne Vaughn. Firebrand Books: Ithaca, NY, 1987. *We Are Everywhere: Writings by and about Lesbian Parents*, edited by Harriet Alpert. The Crossing Press: Freedom, CA, 1988.
Two essential books for any lesbian considering getting pregnant. They give a voice to lesbians from all walks of life, including lesbian co-parents; lesbians who decide not to have children, who adopt or are foster parents; lesbians in heterosexual marriages; lesbians who have their children taken from them or who feel it necessary to give them up; lesbians who were mothers before they were lesbians; and lesbians who are choosing to become parents.

Lesbian and Gay Foster and Adoptive Parents Network
c/o London Friend
86 Caledonian Road
London N1
This is a support group for lesbians and gays who are considering, or are in the process of, adopting or fostering children. They have prepared a pack which includes a list of fostering and adoption agencies, a book list, an article entitled 'Fit for a Family' and the group's aims.

## Books for children

*Asha's Mums*, by Rosamund Elwin and Michele Paulse, illustrated by Dawn Lee. Women's Press: Toronto, 1990.
The message is the same as in *Heather Has Two Mommies* but at least there is a story line and a certain amount of dramatic tension. Asha is a black girl who has to deal with homophobia in her classroom. It is suitable for beginning readers as the print is large and the language not too difficult.

*The Duke Who Outlawed Jelly Beans and Other Stories*, by Johnny Valentine, illustrated by Lynette Schmidt. Alyson Wonderland: Boston, 1991.

This is a series of fascinating fairy tales with superb illustrations. All the children have lesbian mothers or gay fathers, but this is put across so naturally that you never feel you are pushing propaganda down your child's throat.

*Gloria Goes to Gay Pride*, by Leslea Newman, illustrated by Russell Crocker. Alyson Wonderland: Boston, 1991.
This book gives a sanitized view of gay solidarity and reads like propaganda.

*Heather Has Two Mommies*, by Leslea Newman, illustrated by Diana Souza. In Other Words Publishing: Northampton, MA, 1989.
Three-year-old Heather lives in the lesbian version of the ideal nuclear family. Despite its preachiness and lack of story line, it is one of the few children's books which show lesbian mothers and mention donor insemination.

## *Screening (HIV and AIDS)*

### READING LIST

'HIV & AIDS – Information for Lesbians', leaflet from The Terrence Higgins Trust.
'HIV & AIDS – Information for Women', leaflet from The Terrence Higgins Trust.
'Lesbians, HIV & Safer Sex – Low Risk Isn't No Risk', leaflet from London Lesbian and Gay Switchboard.
'Safer Sex for Gay Men', leaflet from The Terrence Higgins Trust.
*Safer Sex: The Guide for Women Today*, by Diane Richardson. Pandora Press: London, 1990.
'Women and HIV and AIDS', leaflet from Women's Health.
*Women and AIDS – an International Resource Book*, by Marge Berer. Pandora Press: London, 1993.

## RESOURCES

**BHAN**
(Black HIV/AIDS Network)
First floor, St Stephen's House
41 Uxbridge Road
Shepherd's Bush
London W12 8LH
Tel. 081–749 2828
Counselling, advice and support
for black people living with or
affected by HIV and AIDS.

**Blackliners**
Unit 46, Eurolink Business Centre
49 Effra Road
London SW12 1BZ
Tel. 071–738 5274 (Mon–Fri
10 a.m.–8.30 p.m.;
Sat 1–6 p.m.)
Helpline for black and Asian
communities affected by HIV/AIDS.

**Mainliners Ltd**
205 Stockwell Road
London SW9 9SL
Tel. 071–737 3141
(10 a.m.–5 p.m. daily)
Support services for those with
HIV/AIDS who are former or
current drug users. Drop-in plus
helpline.

**National AIDS Helpline**
Tel. 0800–567 123
Free, 24-hour confidential phone
line.

**Positively Women**
5 Sebastian St
London EC1V 0HE
Tel. 071–490 5515 and
071–490 2327 (Helpline 12
noon–2 p.m. daily, Mon–Fri)
For all women who have HIV or
AIDS. National support,
counselling and information.

**Terrence Higgins Trust**
52/54 Grays Inn Road
London WC1X 8JU
Tel. 071–242 1010 (Helpline
daily 12 noon–10 p.m.)
071–831 0330 (administration
and advice centre)
Offers wide range of services and
support for all affected by HIV/
AIDS. There is a women's officer
and specifically lesbian counselling
is available.

## Screening (genetic screening)

**Cystic Fibrosis Research Trust**
5 Blyth Road
Bromley, Kent BR1 3RS
Tel. 081–464 7211

**Sickle Cell Society**
54 Station Road
London NW10 4UA
Tel. 081–961 7795

**Tay-Sachs Testing Centre**
Genetics Department
Guy's Hospital
London SE1
Tel. 071–955 4648

**United Kingdom Thalassaemia
Society**
107 Nightingale Lane
London N8 7QY
Tel. 081–348 0437

## Screening (sexual health for women)

The Audre Lorde Clinic
The Ambrose King Centre
The Royal London Hospital
Whitechapel
London E1 1BB
For appointments phone
071–377 7312.
Friday mornings, 9.15 a.m.–
12.30 p.m.
Open to all lesbians for screening
for sexually transmitted infections,
cervical smears, advice and
counselling on sexual matters, free
dental dams, HIV testing, breast
examination.

The Bernhard Clinic
GU Medicine
Charing Cross Hospital
Fulham Palace Road
Hammersmith
London W6 8RF
Tel. 081–846 7606

Wednesday afternoons by
appointment.
Open to all lesbians for screening
for sexually transmitted infections,
cervical smears, advice and
counselling on sexual matters,
breast examination, HIV testing.

## Donor insemination through clinics

Human Fertilisation and
Embryology Authority
Paxton House
30 Artillery Lane
London E1 7LS
Tel. 071–377 5077
Has list of donor insemination
clinics in Britain.

PAS (Pregnancy Advisory Service)
11–13 Charlotte St
London W1P 1HD
Tel. 071–637 8962
Clinic offering donor insemination
service to lesbians and single
women.

*For legal information regarding
women's rights and self-
insemination, readers in the United
States can contact:*

Center for Reproductive Law
and Policy
120 Wall Street
New York, NY 10005
Tel. (212) 514–5534
Fax (212) 514–5538

National Women's Health
Network
1325 G Street NW
Washington DC 20005
Tel. (202) 347–1140

Readers on the West Coast may contact:

Womancare – A Feminist
Health Center
688 Hollister Street, #B
San Diego, CA 92154
Tel. (619) 424–9944
Womancare has run a woman-controlled conception programme since 1984. Its philosophy emphasizes women taking control of their bodies and their lives and firmly recognizes 'the right of all women to choose when, how and whether or not to have children'.

## Getting pregnant

*Getting Pregnant*, by Robert Winston. Anaya Publishers: London, 1989.
Although written for heterosexual couples, this book gives good, clear information on how to get pregnant. It includes an informative chapter evaluating sex-selection methods.

*A Manual of Natural Family Planning*, by Dr Anna M. Flynn and Melissa Brooks. George Allen & Unwin: London, 1988.
An introduction to natural family planning methods for heterosexual couples, which does give useful information on learning how to determine your fertile days.

*Natural Birth Control*, by Katia and Jonathon Drake. Thorson: London, 1987.

## When SI isn't working

*Infertility: What Causes It and What Can Be Done About It*, leaflet from Women's Health. Send 40p plus large 28p stamped SAE.

*In Search of Parenthood – Coping with Infertility and High-tech Conception* by Judith Lasker and Susan Borg. Pandora Press: London, 1989.
An informative and compassionate inside look at the ways in which the new reproductive technologies affect women and men.

*Trying to Have a Baby? Overcoming Infertility and Child Loss*, by Maggie Jones. Sheldon Press: London, 1984.
This book focuses on a woman's reactions to infertility and losing a baby through miscarriage or stillbirth. It has an excellent chapter on the problem of waiting and adapting to childlessness. It is not the best source on the causes and cures of infertility.

## The law

*Lesbian Mothers' Legal Handbook*, by Rights of Women Lesbian Custody Group. The Women's Press: London, 1986. Available from Rights of Women, 52 Featherstone St, London EC1Y 8RT, with 1992 update on

changes in the law.
This book talks about the precautions to take if lesbians want to keep charge of their children, and what to do if they find themselves in a custody dispute. It gives practical information on immigration, police arrest, making a will, adoption and fostering, legal aid and custody law.

'Lesbian mothers, lesbian families: Legal obstacles, legal challenges', by Nancy Polikoff, in *Politics of the Heart – A Lesbian Parenting Anthology*, edited by Sandra Pollack and Jeanne Vaughn. Firebrand Books: New York, 1987.
This article raises the political issues for lesbians of fighting for legal recognition of lesbian families.

Lesbian Custody Project,
Rights of Women
52 Featherstone St
London EC1Y 8RT
Tel. 071–251 6577
Information, leaflets and legal advice for lesbian mothers.

Campaign Against The Child Support Act
King's Cross Women's Centre
71 Tonbridge St
London WC1H 9DZ
Tel. London, 071–837 7509;
Bristol, 0272–426 608;
Manchester, 061–344 0758.
Information, leaflets, petitions and

advice on individual cases. The Campaign is coordinated by the Wages for Housework Campaign and Payday men's network.

If you have trouble ordering these books through your local library or bookshop, try:
Silver Moon Bookshop
68 Charing Cross Road
London WC2
Tel. 071–836 7906

# *Advice for Donors about Self-insemination*

THIS leaflet is a summary of what self-insemination is all about and what you will be asked to do if you agree to be a donor. It is not aimed at men who have been asked to co-parent.

Your contribution and cooperation would be greatly appreciated. Without such help, lesbians and single women have a very hard time getting pregnant, as most donor-insemination clinics are biased in favour of heterosexual couples. However, think seriously before you agree, and do not be a donor if you feel at all uneasy. You need to think about how you might feel knowing that you had fathered a child or if you were contacted one day by the child. Some very young children ask to see their donors, and their mothers may want to arrange this. Or the child might be a teenager or young adult before deciding to trace you. How would you feel about this?

## Donor – not father

You are being asked to donate your sperm to a woman who will be raising the child either on her own or with a lesbian partner, without a man as father. You are doing this on the understanding that you will not insist on parental responsibility for the child that results. You will not be asked to act as a father or pay any maintenance or have any parental obligations towards the child. You may be asked if you are willing to be contacted if the child wants to meet its genetic father.

## Screening for health

You should be free of sexually transmitted diseases, be willing to have an HIV test, be practising safer sex and/or be able to reassure the woman that you have not been doing anything which puts you at risk of HIV infection. You may be asked intimate questions about your sex life, which must be answered honestly so that the woman can assess whether she is putting herself or her baby at risk by using your semen. You may also be asked about genetic conditions in you or your family which could be passed on. You may be asked to fill in a medical questionnaire.

## Donating the sperm

Simply masturbate and ejaculate into a clean jar, preferably plastic. Styrofoam and condoms are not recommended because they may harm the sperm. The pot need not be sterile but should be well washed and rinsed of all traces of detergent.

You need not abstain from sexual activity before inseminations. It's a myth that abstaining from ejaculation for two or three days will improve the sperm count or strengthen the sperm in any way. Sexual activity in general increases sperm production. You will have a higher sperm count if you ejaculate a few days before the woman's first insemination. Your sperm count may be affected by antibiotics. If you take antibiotics in the 70 days before the insemination, tell the woman about it.

If there is a delay before you can hand the semen to the woman, keep it at room temperature or body temperature (next to your skin) but certainly not any warmer. Heating the sperm by placing the jar in front of a fire or in direct sunlight will kill them.

## Being available

A woman is fertile for a few days (2–7) during her menstrual cycle. The fertile days are those in which she is potentially able to get pregnant and during which she will want to inseminate.

It is not possible to predict much in advance when these fertile days will be. The woman can give you a rough idea what week she might be fertile in, but will have to contact you nearer the time to arrange the best days. This means it is very important that you are flexible and easy to contact.

## How long should it take for her to conceive?

It is, of course, possible for her to conceive after only one insemination, but don't count on it. Be prepared to be donating for several months to a year before she gets pregnant. You will maximize her chances of getting pregnant by doing at least two and preferably three to five inseminations in each cycle. The more often you do the inseminations within the fertile part of her cycle, the more likely she is to become pregnant sooner.

## Finding out more

If you want to know more, you can read *Challenging Conceptions: Pregnancy and Parenting Beyond the Traditional Family*, by Lisa Saffron, published by Cassell, London, 1994. The book includes accounts of the experiences of several men who have been donors.

# Questionnaire for Donors

## Personal details

Name ...............................................................................................................................

Address ...........................................................................................................................

.........................................................................................................................................

.........................................................................................................................................

Phone number ..................................... Date of birth..............................................

Height ................................................. Weight ......................................................

Hair colour .......................................... Eye colour ................................................

Race/ethnic origin.............................................................................................................

Have you fathered any children? If so, how many?...........................................................

Have you had a recent semen analysis? If so, when, and what was the result? ..................

.........................................................................................................................................

## Medical history

What is your blood group?

   ABO.............................................................

   Rhesus factor .............................................

Do you have any of these sexually transmitted diseases?

   Gonorrhoea ............................................. Syphilis...............................................

   Herpes...................................................... Hepatitis B (serum hepatitis) .............................

   Non-specific urethritis (NSU) .........................................................................................

If you haven't already been, would you be willing to go to an STD clinic to be screened?

When was the last time you had an HIV test?

What was the result?.........................................................................................................

Even if your HIV test was negative, you could still be infected with HIV in the six months before or since the test. For this reason, it is important that you answer the following questions about high-risk activities.

   Are your current sexual partners uninfected? How do you know? .........................................

   .....................................................................................................................................

   Do you:

      Have anal sex without a condom? ........................................................................

      Have vaginal intercourse without a condom?.........................................................

      Use sex toys that could get blood on them? .........................................................

   Do you inject drugs and share injecting equipment? ..........................................................

   Do you  share razors or blades?.......................................................................................

   Have you had any tattoos done or your ears pierced within the last six months? ...................

   Have you ever had a blood transfusion in another country? ................................................

## Fertility

The following activities could affect how fertile you are.

Have you been in an occupation involving a risk of radiation or chemical exposure or had an accident with radioactive or chemical materials? ...........................................

Are you a heavy user of:

alcohol? ...............................................................................................................

drugs (if so, which ones)? ...................................................................................

cigarettes? ..........................................................................................................

Are you taking chronic medication? If so, what kind and what for ...............................

## Genetic conditions

Have you or anyone in your family had any of the following conditions? Consider your family to be brothers, sisters, father, mother, maternal and paternal aunts and uncles and grandparents, including those who have died.

Allergies (such as eczema, asthma, hayfever) .......................

Cirrhosis of the liver (juvenile) ...............................................

| | |
|---|---|
| Cleft palate or lip ................................. | Clubfoot ............................................... |
| Congenital heart disease .................... | Cystic fibrosis ..................................... |
| Deafness before age 50 ...................... | Diabetes (adult-onset) ......................... |
| Glaucoma .............................................. | Heart attack before age 50 .................. |
| Huntington's chorea ............................. | Hydrocephalus ...................................... |
| Hyperlipidaemia .................................... | Kidney disease (early progressive) ........... |
| Neurofibromatosis ................................ | Restricted growth .................................. |
| Spina bifida .......................................... | Stroke before age 50 ............................ |

If yes to any, please say which specific relation had which condition. .......................
..........................................................................................................................
..........................................................................................................................

Are you a carrier of:

| | |
|---|---|
| Thalassaemia? ..................................... | Sickle-cell disease? .............................. |
| Tay-Sachs disease ............................... | Cystic fibrosis? ..................................... |

## Being a donor

Do you agree that you would not claim parental responsibility for any child born from your donation? ......................................................................................................

Over how long a period would you be committed to donating sperm? ...........................

Can you be available when needed, two to six times per month? ..................................

*Fertility Chart*

| Temperature | | |
|---|---|---|
| °F | °C | |
| 99.3 | 37.25 | |
| 99.2 | 37.20 | |
| 99.1 | 37.15 | |
| 99.0° | 37.10 | |
| 98.9 | 37.05 | |
| 98.8 | 37.00 | |
| 98.7 | 36.95 | |
| 98.6 | 36.90 | |
| 98.5 | 36.85 | |
| 98.4 | 36.80 | |
| 98.3 | 36.75 | |
| 98.2 | 36.70 | |
| 98.1 | 36.65 | |
| 98.0 | 36.60 | |
| 97.9 | 36.55 | |
| 97.8 | 36.50 | |
| 97.7 | 36.45 | |
| 97.6 | 36.40 | |
| 97.5 | 36.35 | |
| 97.4 | 36.30 | |
| 97.3 | 36.25 | |
| 97.2 | 36.20 | |
| 97.1 | 36.15 | |
| 97.0 | 36.10 | |
| 96.9 | 36.05 | |
| 96.8 | 36.00 | |
| Date | | |
| Day | | 1 2 3 4 5 6 7 8 9 10 11 12 13 14 15 16 17 1° 19 20 21 22 23 24 25 26 27 28 29 30 31 32 33 34 35 36 37 38 39 40 |

| | | Day | 1 | 2 | 3 | 4 | 5 | 6 | 7 | 8 | 9 | 10 | 11 | 12 | 13 | 14 | 15 | 16 | 17 | 18 | 19 | 20 | 21 | 22 | 23 | 24 | 25 | 26 | 27 | 28 | 29 | 30 | 31 | 32 | 33 | 34 | 35 | 36 | 37 | 38 | 39 | 40 |
|---|---|---|---|---|---|---|---|---|---|---|---|---|---|---|---|---|---|---|---|---|---|---|---|---|---|---|---|---|---|---|---|---|---|---|---|---|---|---|---|---|---|---|
| | | Period/spotting | | | | | | | | | | | | | | | | | | | | | | | | | | | | | | | | | | | | | | | | | |
| Mucus | Sensation | | | | | | | | | | | | | | | | | | | | | | | | | | | | | | | | | | | | | | | | | | |
| | Appearance | | | | | | | | | | | | | | | | | | | | | | | | | | | | | | | | | | | | | | | | | | |
| Cervix | Position | | | | | | | | | | | | | | | | | | | | | | | | | | | | | | | | | | | | | | | | | | |
| | Opening | | | | | | | | | | | | | | | | | | | | | | | | | | | | | | | | | | | | | | | | | | |
| | Firmness | | | | | | | | | | | | | | | | | | | | | | | | | | | | | | | | | | | | | | | | | | |
| | | Pain | | | | | | | | | | | | | | | | | | | | | | | | | | | | | | | | | | | | | | | | | |
| | | Breast tenderness | | | | | | | | | | | | | | | | | | | | | | | | | | | | | | | | | | | | | | | | | |
| | | Disturbances | | | | | | | | | | | | | | | | | | | | | | | | | | | | | | | | | | | | | | | | | |
| | | Fertile days | | | | | | | | | | | | | | | | | | | | | | | | | | | | | | | | | | | | | | | | | |
| | | Insemination | | | | | | | | | | | | | | | | | | | | | | | | | | | | | | | | | | | | | | | | | |
| | | Date | | | | | | | | | | | | | | | | | | | | | | | | | | | | | | | | | | | | | | | | | |

# Index

DISCARD